THE

GL

COOKBOOK
─── AND ───
DIET PLAN

THE GL
COOKBOOK
AND
DIET PLAN

*A Glycemic Load Weight-Loss Program
with Over 150
Delicious Recipes*

NIGEL DENBY

**with Tina Michelucci
& Deborah Pyner**

Ulysses Press

Published in the United States by
ULYSSES PRESS
P.O. Box 3440
Berkeley, CA 94703
www.ulyssespress.com

First published as *The GL Diet Cookbook* in the U.K. in 2006
by HarperThorsons, an imprint of HarperCollins*Publishers*

ISBN10: 1-56975-611-2
ISBN13: 978-1-56975-611-9
Library of Congress Catalog Number: 2006938937

1 3 5 7 9 10 8 6 4 2

Printed in Canada by Transcontinental Printing

U.S. Proofreader: Tiffany Watson
U.S. Editorial & Production: Tamara Kowalski, Ruth Marcus,
Matt Orendorff, Elyce Petker, Laurel Shane
Cover design: Double R Design

Distributed by Publishers Group West

This publication is meant to be used as a general reference and recipe book to aid weight
loss. As with any weight-loss plan, before commencing we would strongly recommend that
you consult your doctor to see whether it is suitable for you.

The publishers, authors, or Diet Freedom Limited, directly or indirectly, do not
dispense medical advice.

While all reasonable care has been taken during the preparation of this book, the
publishers, editors and authors cannot accept responsibility for any
consequences arising from the use of this information.

This book includes reference to nuts and recipes including nuts, nut derivatives and nut oils.
Avoid if you have a known allergic reaction. Pregnant and nursing mothers,
invalids, the elderly, children and babies may be potentially vulnerable to nut
allergies and should therefore avoid nuts, nut derivatives and nut oils.

ß

Contents

Acknowledgments

A huge thank you to our ever-increasing band of Diet Freedom supporters, gathered from our previous books, *The 7-Day GL Diet* and *The GL Diet*, our website, www.dietfreedom.co.uk, and by word of mouth. It is your support that continues to motivate us to do better, and help you to the best of our ability in achieving your goals. Your honesty and feedback are invaluable and much admired.

Last but not least, not forgetting our wonderful partners, families and friends who have been unwavering in their support of our working hours and our passion in getting things right, even when we are painful to live with!

Thank you so much.

Lots of love,

Tina, Deborah and Nigel
xxx

Introduction

There is little doubt that in recent years the principles of low-glycemic eating have gathered more and more support from dieticians, doctors and health organizations such as Diabetes UK and leading heart health and cancer charities.

The concept of being able to determine a food's effect on blood sugars has been described as "the most significant nutritional development for 50 years" and has been conclusively shown to be a solution to a lifetime of yo-yo dieting for millions of people.

Unlike so many other weight-loss plans, the low-glycemic approach is well respected as not only an effective weight-control tool but also for a host of health benefits, including reduced risk of heart disease, diabetes, high blood pressure and some cancers.

The Glycemic Index (GI), which is the basis of low-glycemic diets, is not a new idea. It has been researched and developed at major universities around the world for the past 25 years, but only really hit the mainstream a few years ago.

As with all science, nutrition is constantly evolving. What started as a complicated (and in some cases inaccurate) way of classifying carbohydrate-containing foods, the Glycemic Index (GI) has been developed into a simpler, more accurate, user-friendly system in the Glycemic Load (GL).

The Glycemic Index classifies some foods we know to be inherently "healthy" as being foods we should avoid. It also suggests other foods can be eaten freely, when in fact they may have a detrimental effect on our all-important blood sugars—why the inconsistency?

Simple—the Glycemic Index is a laboratory test which requires that *specific amounts* of different foods are tested in order to produce comparable results. The Glycemic Index doesn't take into account the amount of food we actually eat, and so the Index on its own can be misleading and confusing.

The Glycemic Load removes these confusions and inaccuracies. It means more food choices and less room for error.

Having used the GL principles with my patients for some years now in my clinics, what I can tell you is that using the GL is the most effective weight-loss tool I have seen in my career, and the results achieved and feedback from our Diet Freedom Club Members online at www.dietfreedom.co.uk has reinforced this tenfold.

My patients, our readers and our Diet Freedom Club Members get results, maintain them, and tell us that for the first time in years they feel free of the "diet trap" and able to get on with their lives. They feel well, have more energy and rediscover a long-lost optimistic outlook on life—something they have been missing for years. What more could we ask of an eating plan?

The principle of the GL diet is simple: Stable blood sugars means less excess energy stored as fat and fewer food cravings. We have been very careful in our previous books (*The GL Diet* and *The 7-Day GL Diet*), as in this cookbook, to ensure that our recipes and advice tick *all* the healthy eating boxes.

As well as eating low-GL foods, we advocate good fats, no added salt wherever possible, plenty of fruit and vegetables and good-quality proteins including fish, lean meats and poultry, beans and, of course, a good dose of physical activity—not "exercise"—we don't like that word—no, it's got to be **A C T I V I T Y** and it's got to be fun!

This isn't a here-today, gone-tomorrow fad diet. I wouldn't put my name to it if it were. This is a way of eating you can adopt for life, and it is very satisfying to see that more and more people are finding it offers them what no other diet has before: results and, more important, results they can maintain forever.

What we've done with this cookbook is make an already simple principle even easier. You don't have to do any boring counting (who has the time?!) or weighing of foods (unless you want to), and there is absolutely no need to be hungry—so don't worry, you won't be.

So what a low-GL diet DOES mean is delicious food you'll love, food that loves you back, and heaps of variety to make sure you get all the nutritional goodies you need.

It also means "time freedom." If you are as busy as most of us, you probably won't want to come home after a tiring day and start preparing a whole host of weird and wonderful ingredients before you can even start cooking! Tina and Deborah have made sure that they have included lots of quick and easy recipes with this in mind.

We've designed a simple low-GL template for your guidance so that you can slot in whatever recipes you fancy. Choose from our "fast and friendly" selection for quick, throw-together no-nonsense cooking, or from the host of veggie-friendly recipes. Our vegetarian friends are so often forgotten when it comes to diets, so we've taken some interesting ingredients to give you anything but the normal humdrum veggie selection.

And then, for when you have the time and inclination and feel like pushing the boat out a bit, we've got some delicious foodie-friendly recipes for keen cooks. Maybe you fancy a lazy breakfast and have a bit more time to prepare it, or you have friends or family over for dinner? We at Diet Freedom HQ love food and get a real buzz out of preparing good food for the people we love, so we hope you'll find the foodie-friendly recipes great for those special occasions.

Bon appétit!

Nigel Denby
Registered Dietician
RD BSc Hons

Chapter 1

HOW TO USE THIS BOOK

First and foremost we want you to enjoy this cookbook.

The last thing we want is for you to get hung up about working out or counting up the GL scores of foods, or weighing out every ingredient, so don't do any of that. Counting is boring and stressful and can lead to overeating in itself. We have provided the estimated GL scores of the recipes, but only as a guide.

The basis of all the recipes is that we have swapped high-GL ingredients for low-GL ones. So if the recipe contains carbs, we have replaced the FAST carbs with SLOW ones.

We've also put together all the other pieces of the "healthy eating jigsaw" to make sure that your low-GL diet is nicely balanced and full of lots of good, healthy and nutritious foods.

Rather than giving you very prescriptive plans and menus ("you must eat this today for breakfast and that for lunch tomorrow"), we've given you a basic template to help you plan your own low-GL healthy eating a week at a time. The template will help you make sure you eat regularly, eat a good variety of foods and, of course, choose the foods you love.

Now, because we've done everything we can think of to make using this cookbook as easy as possible, we want you to do something for us. We want you to "think natural" and try, wherever possible, to start with basic ingredients, follow a few simple steps and end up with a delicious, natural, healthy dish. We're talking about cooking from scratch, not fancy *cordon bleu* stuff, just simple "back to basics" cooking.

We are passionate about cutting back on highly processed foods because they can be full of hidden sugars, salt, additives and unhealthy trans fats. The bottom line with all of our recipes is that you start with a bunch of natural ingredients and combine them together. This means you are in total control over what you consume, with no hidden "nasties" to worry about. We have also given you lots of short-cuts to help save you time and effort, without compromising on any of the health and taste benefits.

Weight Loss and A Whole Lot More

Low GL is about a lot more than weight loss. That's why more and more national and international health organizations are joining together to recommend a low-GL diet as the most appropriate for good health. Diabetes, high blood pressure, heart disease, some cancers and the symptoms of hormonal disturbances like Polycystic Ovarian Syndrome (PCOS), premenstrual syndrome (PMS) and menopause can all be prevented or eased by a low-GL diet.

Let's Get Down to Basics

OK, so now that we know why following a low-GL diet is so good for weight control and general health, let's get on with it! The basic templates (pages 15 and 19) will help you with balanced menu planning and shopping. We've based the templates on the basic principles of a healthy, balanced diet.

For instance, most of us know we should eat some oily fish every week, have five portions of fruit and vegetables every day and include dairy foods, which are a good source of calcium for healthy bones. The templates show you how to organize healthy low-GL eating by thinking about your day, deciding how much time you've got to prepare food, whether you'll be eating on the run or eating out, and balancing your foods throughout the day. If you have meat for lunch, you probably don't need meat again for dinner. Or if you struggle to eat a substantial breakfast, make sure you have a decent mid-morning snack to help you stay in the driving seat till lunch time.

The templates will give you the confidence to know that you are not only lowering your overall glycemic load (GL) but also eating a good balance of food and nutrients at the same time.

The Principles of Healthy Eating

	Daily and weekly	Tips
Alcohol	1 unit = ½ glass of wine ½ pint of regular strength beer, cider or lager 1 shot of spirits Men—weekly intake < 21 units, with at least 3 alcohol-free days. Women—weekly intake < 14 units with at least 3 alcohol-free days.	If you do indulge, go for a glass of wine watered down with soda or sparkling mineral water.
Dairy	3 portions a day. Milk on cereal, a matchbox-size piece of cheese or a small tub of yogurt all count as 1 portion. If in weight-loss mode, we recommend up to a glass of milk per day and no more than 2.5oz low-fat or 1.7oz high-fat cheese per day.	If you don't eat dairy foods remember to make sure you choose calcium-enriched non-dairy alternatives such as soy (look for no-added-sugar versions). You can use any milk you prefer but if you are concerned about your overall fat intake use skim or lowfat
Eggs	1 a day	

	Daily and weekly	Tips
Fiber	4–5 servings (around 18g) fiber-rich foods every day	Soluble fiber = oats, fruits, beans. Insoluble fiber = vegetables, whole grains, cereals
Fluid	1½–2 liters a day	Can include tea or coffee (try to limit to 3 cups total), diluted fruit/vegetable juice, herb and fruit teas and water. Alcohol does not count!
Fruit and Vegetables	5 a day—choose as many different colors as possible, and try to divide equally between fruits and vegetables. A "portion" is generally considered to be 80g.	1 piece of fruit or glass of juice with added water at breakfast. A piece of fruit mid-morning. Some salad or vegetable soup at lunch and 2 portions of vegetables or salad with dinner and you've done it!
Meat	Fresh, good-quality lean meat such as chicken and turkey. Buy organic wherever possible.	Try to keep to a maximum of 3 portions of red meat per week.

	Daily and weekly	**Tips**
Nuts and seeds	Choose unsalted varieties and go for a good mixture of both nuts and seeds.	A small handful a day (as a snack or in salads or muesli) will give you a great nutrient boost and has been shown to help keep hunger at bay.
Oily fish	Aim for 1–2 portions a week of salmon, trout, sardines, mackerel, fresh tuna, pilchards, herring, rainbow trout or other dark oily fish.	If you don't eat fish, flax seeds or omega 3-enriched eggs are good ways of getting your essential fatty acids.
Beans	3 portions a week in the form of chickpeas, beans (butter beans, garbanzo beans, low-sugar bakes beans, etc.) and lentils	Add beans to soups and recipes. Puréed beans, seasoned with herbs and spices, make great dips and spreads. Keep cans of (no-sugar-added) chickpeas or other beans on hand for a snack. Rinse and drain, then blend with cumin, garlic, tahini (sesame seed paste) or olive oil and lemon juice for a speedy, healthy dip.

	Daily and weekly	**Tips**
Salt	Aim to limit salt to a maximum of 6 grams a day or less.	Reduce the amount of processed food you eat, and don't add salt during cooking or at the table.
Saturated fat (within the TOTAL fat amount below)	Men—aim to limit total saturated fat intake to 30g a day Women—20g a day.	Trim visible fat from meats and remove skin from poultry. Use lower-fat milk and dairy foods. Minimize butter and cream. Use olive oil–based spread instead of butter.
Total fat	Men—aim to limit total fat intake to 95g a day Women—70g a day	Work on reducing the amount of fats and oils you add when cooking. Don't eat deep-fried foods.

Can I Follow the GL Diet if I'm Vegetarian?

Vegetarians can follow the same healthy low-GL principles as meat-eaters, choosing foods from each of the major food groups, high-protein sources, cereals and grains, dairy products (or soy substitutes), vegetables and fruits. Obviously the more restrictive the diet, the more difficult it becomes to ensure all the body's nutritional requirements are being met. Deciding to follow a vegetarian diet means ensuring that nutrients usually provided by meat or dairy products are obtained from other foods. With some careful consideration, this is easily done.

Calcium

Aim to include three servings of dairy per day. If you don't eat dairy products, choose calcium-enriched soy or tofu, dried fruits such as apricots, green leafy vegetables and nuts and seeds to help meet your calcium requirements.

Iron

Non-meat eaters have to be careful about their iron levels, since the type of iron found in red meat is particularly well absorbed in the body. Other sources of iron include bread, beans, green leafy vegetables and dried fruits.

Protein

Vegetarians substitute meat with other protein foods such as beans (lentils, chickpeas and beans), dairy products, eggs and nuts. If you don't eat dairy foods, soy, tofu and Quorn are good protein alternatives.

Vitamin B12

People who exclude all animal products from their diet may develop a deficiency of vitamin B12, so they should take a good-quality multi-vitamin and mineral supplement that includes it, as this vitamin does not occur naturally in plant-based foods.

Zinc

Meat and dairy products are rich sources of zinc, and if you don't eat these you may wish to consider a good quality multivitamin and mineral supplement which includes it.

Main Points to Remember

- Enjoy your food—if you don't like it, don't eat it!
- Eat regularly—every 4 hours is a good guide. Don't skip meals or snacks—you are almost certain to pay for it by overeating or making poor food choices later.
- Eat a good variety of foods—try new things—there are so many fabulous foods out there!
- Get "slow-carb savvy" and learn to swap high-GL foods for low-GL ones (see page 80).
- Keep hydrated—remember to get 1½–2 liters of fluid a day.
- Try to avoid food with added sugar, glucose, glucose syrups and high fructose corn syrups (not to be confused with fructose). Get your sweetness from fruits and the occasional piece of high-cocoa dark chocolate (70 percent or more cocoa). Sweeten recipes with natural agave syrup or fructose.
- A lapse is just a lapse, don't turn it into a relapse!

Memory Box

- Eat every 4 hours
- 5-a-day fruit and vegetables
- Avoid added sugar
- Avoid added salt
- Minimum 1½ liters of fluid a day
- Eat at least one portion of oily fish a week
- Eat a good variety of protein foods
- Cut right down on the booze!

A Week's Worth of Tips

Read through the tips below to help you get on the right track, then check out the sample weekly plans (pages 15 and 19, and you can also print these from our website, www.dietfreedom.co.uk) to help you manage your weekly food intake.

Breakfast

- Keep a batch of muesli made up for when you are in a hurry.
- Not very hungry? Have a smoothie—a great way of getting some fruit and dairy portions into the day.
- Have a small glass of fruit juice topped up with water if you're struggling with getting your 5-a-day fruit and vegetables.

- How about some good old-fashioned oatmeal?
- Choose something yogurt-based—a small portion of yogurt is 1 of your 3 daily dairy portions for healthy bones.
- Got a bit more time to spare today? Treat yourself to a healthy cooked breakfast (see page 142).
- Feeling decadent? Smoked salmon counts as a portion of heart-friendly oily fish. How about a lazy breakfast of smoked salmon, eggs and rye toast? (See page 165.)

Mid-Morning Snack

- Keep forgetting to have your snacks? Use your mobile, palm pilot or email to send yourself a reminder.
- After a lighter breakfast, a more substantial snack like a couple of oat cakes and some hummus or smoked fish paté will fit the bill.
- Some crudités and a yogurt or hummus dip will count as 1 of your 5 fruit and vegetables for the day.
- Got a craving for something sweet? Try 4–5 dried apricots.
- Next time you go to the bathroom check the color of your urine—if it's darker than straw, you are not drinking enough water.
- If you miss your snack, you are far more likely to end up in the biscuit barrel or at the vending machine.
- Hey! Don't forget you can eat chocolate! Choose a small portion (2 squares) of dark chocolate with 70 percent or more cocoa solids.
- Mixed toasted seeds are delicious and nutritious!

Lunch

■ How about chickpea salad (page 216) to get 1 of your 3 portions of beans a week?

■ If you're going for something with pasta, remember cooking it *al dente* helps keep the GL lower.

■ Don't forget, you don't need to add salt to your food. Use the guide to using herbs and spices in Chapter 5.

■ Sandwich on the run? Make it an open one to keep the GL low.

■ Never made your own soup? Try our recipe for "No-fuss Lentil Soup" (page 130)—it's quick to prepare and tastes divine!

■ Friends coming round for lunch? Why not whip up a healthy low-GL soup such as the fennel soup on page 124?

■ Family roast? No problem, check out our recipes on pages 192–5.

Mid-Afternoon Snack

■ A matchbox-size piece of cheese counts as 1 of your 3 portions of dairy foods a day.

■ Keep a bowl of fruit on your desk—if it's under your nose you're more likely to eat it!

■ A handful of unsalted nuts has been shown to reduce hunger later in the day.

■ Guacamole makes a great topping on an oatcake or rye cracker, and counts as another portion of vegetable.

- Cottage cheese is a great dairy source and tastes delicious with fresh pineapple or mango.
- How's that fruit bowl looking? About ready for topping up?
- Getting fed up with oat cakes? Try rye crispbreads such as Ryvita with some sugar-free peanut butter for a change.

Dinner

- Fancy something fishy? A 4 g portion of oily fish counts as one of your 2 portions for the week.
- If you are going to struggle to get time to make lunch tomorrow, make a little extra tonight so you've got some leftovers. The Crustless Spinach Tart (page 186) is great for this.
- When you're choosing meats, select the leanest cuts and ask for any visible fat to be trimmed.
- Out to dinner tonight? Make sure you have all your meals and snacks today, and order a large glass of water to sip while you look at the menu—trust us, it really helps!
- When shopping for fruit and vegetables choose as many different colors as possible to get the best mix of protective antioxidants—"Eat a rainbow" every day!
- Fancy rice tonight? Try pearl barley as an alternative, or mix some lentils with the lower-GL brown or wild rice.
- We all like the odd night chilling in front of the TV. Try our Pork with Mustard Sauce and Pasta dish on page 116.

Sample Weekly Plan for Meat-eaters

This is to give you an idea of how to put together a healthy low-GL week.

*Where the following are mentioned in the sample plans below, recommended portion sizes are –

- MEN: oatcakes/crispbreads up to 4, bread up to 2 slices
- WOMEN: oatcakes/crispbreads up to 2, bread 1 slice

	Day 1	Day 2	Day 3	Day 4	Day 5	Day 6	Day 7
Breakfast	Melon & orange smoothie (page 95)	Zesty yog-bowl (page 147)	Poached eggs on toast	Orange spice oatmeal (page 140)	Coconut & apricot energy shake (page 101)	Mushroom "toast," scrambled egg & bacon (page 142)	Smoked salmon & eggs with rye toast (page 165)
Mid-morning Snack	Oatcakes with cream cheese and cucumber	1 apple	Small handful of toasted seeds	1 pear	Small handful of unsalted nuts	1 orange/ tangerine	Small handful of cherries or grapes
Lunch	Broccoli & almond soup (page 106)	Perky egg & asparagus (page 107)	Hot dressed salad (page 149)	Pumpkin & coconut soup (page 104)	Shrimp cocktail wrap (page 222)	Walnut & goat's cheese salad (page 212)	Roast chicken gorgonzola (page 193)

	Day 1	Day 2	Day 3	Day 4	Day 5	Day 6	Day 7
Mid-afternoon Snack	Small handful of dried apricots	Small handful of toasted seeds	Small handful of dried cranberries (sugar free)	1 tub of cottage cheese	Matchbox-sized piece of cheese	Oatcakes with hummus	1 peach
Dinner	Tuna steak with butter beans (page 114)	Steak, mushroom & red pepper stir-fry (page 115)	Salmon & tomato with lime sauce (page 112)	Chickpea salad (page 216)	One-pot pork & orange casserole (page 169)	Roast turkey (page 192)	Fennel soup (page 124)

Sample Weekly Plan for Vegetarians

This is to give you an idea of how to put together a healthy, low-GL week.

	Day 1	Day 2	Day 3	Day 4	Day 5	Day 6	Day 7
Breakfast	"Feelin' fruity" yog-bowl (page 117)	Banana and strawberry smoothie (page 118)	Apple & hazelnut muesli (page 119)	Apricot & almond smoothie (page 120)	Pear & pumpkin seed yog-bowl (page 121)	Tofu & sunflower smoothie (page 122)	Hot apple oatmeal (page 123)
Mid-morning Snack	Small handful of toasted seeds	Oatcakes with sugar-free peanut butter	1 apple	Carrot batons with sour cream and chive dip	Small handful of cherries	Celery sticks with hummus dip	Choco craving drink (page 226)
Lunch	Chicory with watercress & orange (page 125)	Spinach, avocado, pea & mint salad (page 126)	Grilled asparagus with feta cheese (page 127)	No-fuss lentil soup (page 130)	Spinach & cheese soufflé (page 128)	Spicy aduki bean soup (page 131)	Beanie casserole (page 138)

	Day 1	Day 2	Day 3	Day 4	Day 5	Day 6	Day 7
Mid-afternoon Snack	Small handful of grapes	Matchbox-size piece of cheese	Small handful of dried apricots	Small container of cottage cheese	Oatcakes with red pepper paté	1 pear	Avocado hummus with cucumber sticks
Dinner	Spicy tofu (page 132)	Spicy vegetable dhal (page 136)	Eastern vegetables (page 133)	Hot vegetable stir-fry with coconut milk (page 134)	Bulgur and butternut squash (page 137)	Cheese and mushroom tortilla (page 139)	Grilled veggie wrap (page 221)

Now It's Your Turn!

Once you have read the book thoroughly, including the healthy eating guidelines, and looked through the recipes and snack ideas to see which appeal to you, you are ready to fill in your first low-GL week!

Use a pencil so you can reuse the blank template on page 284. Don't worry, you don't have to fill this in every week (!) but it's a great exercise to get you thinking about a balanced low-GL diet. It will help you to start to "think low GL."

Obviously, most of us don't have the time or inclination to make up recipes for all meals—so use quick, healthy alternatives whenever you wish, again based on the guidelines throughout the book.

Chapter 2

WHAT AFFECTS A FOOD'S GL?

Portion Size

To calculate the GL of a food you need three pieces of information:

- The tested GI of the food
- The portion size
- The number of grams of carbs in the portion.

You then simply divide the GI number by 100, then multiply that figure by the number of grams of carbs in the portion.

Example

If a food has a tested GI of 50 and a 100g portion contains 10 grams of carbs:

50 divided by 100 = 0.5
0.5 x 10 carbs = a GL of 5

If you eat two 100-g portions of that food, the GL would double to 10.

- 10 GL or less is classed as low
- 11–19 GL is medium
- 20+ GL is high

The GL is a far more accurate reference than the GI alone, because it takes into account a food's tested GI response in the body plus the size of the portion *and* how many carbs are in that portion. So it combines the quality of the carb as well as the quantity to give you the whole picture instead of just part of it.

The GI of a food is the same whether you eat one portion or 10 (!), which makes it difficult to use as a weight-loss tool as it is completely unrelated to portion sizes—a key factor for weight loss and health.

Portions are SO important—even when using the GL—so remember that just because 100g of a specific food has a low GL of 5, if you eat three portions of it the GL becomes 15 (i.e. moderate).

By understanding the GL of foods and choosing mainly low-GL foods, you can eat more food overall in quantity—BUT it's still not a license to go bananas!

Food Processing

The way a food is processed affects its GL considerably.

Generally speaking, the more processed, the higher the GL. The nearer a food is to its natural state, the lower the GL.

Bread is a good example—the highly refined and processed, fluffy white breads have a higher GL than the whole grain, darker dense breads.

The whole grains in whole grain bread slow down the digestive process, so we can say it is a SLOW carb food, whereas white refined breads are digested much more quickly, producing a sharp rise in blood glucose. We call foods like this FAST carbs.

Similarly, the GL of an apple is low—but if you remove the peel, which contains a lot of fiber, and process it into a concentrated apple juice, the GL rises.

Food Additives

There are many E numbers and enzymes added to foods during processing, either to enhance taste or texture and/or to prolong shelf-life.

We don't know yet exactly how each of these additives affect the GL, but chances are they have an impact, so again, the less tampered with a food is, the better. If a food label starts to sound like a chemistry lesson ... our advice is to leave it on the shelf!

Cooking Methods and Times

The GL has been shown to rise after a food is cooked, which makes sense as the food will generally become softer and more easily digested, meaning it will break down into glucose more quickly once eaten, causing a faster rise in blood sugar levels.

Pasta is a good example. If you cook it until it's *al dente* (firm to the bite), the GL will be lower than if you cook it until it is soft.

Raw food is best wherever possible and safe. If you have to heat it, do so gently and don't boil the life out of it or burn it to a crisp!

Ripeness and the Age of a Food

The more ripe or aged a food becomes, the more starches and sugars are released, so it makes sense that a new, baby potato has a lower GL than a large baking potato, and that a ripe banana has a higher GL than an under-ripe one.

Eat baby vegetables when possible, and fruits when slightly under-ripe rather than over-ripe to help keep your GL score as low as possible for the day.

Adding Acidity

Tests have shown that if you add acidity such as lemon juice or vinegar to a high-carb meal it can lower the glycemic response by up to 30 percent. This is believed to be because acid slows stomach-emptying and therefore the rate of digestion.

Red wine vinegar and lemon juice have been shown to have the greatest effect when added to foods. It is thought that the body's low-glycemic response to yogurt and sourdough breads is due to their high acidity.

Another good reason to use vinegar is that researchers in Sweden have found that vinegar may help us to eat less and reduce the cravings induced by blood-sugar spikes after meals. Interestingly, they found a direct link between increased vinegar intake and satiety (feelings of fullness and satisfaction) after eating.

So, no excuses, get those fresh lemons and vinegars out, add some olive oil and start making a GL-lowering concoction ... and no, before you ask, this doesn't mean that you can now eat fries floating in vinegar with impunity!

Fiber Content

There are two types of fiber—soluble and insoluble.

Insoluble fiber helps move bulk through the intestine, which together with fluid and being active helps relieve constipation and has been linked with a reduction in the incidence of colon cancers.

Vegetables and many fruits and root vegetables contain fiber only in their skins, so try not to remove them wherever possible.

When insoluble fiber is finely milled and processed it allows enzymes to cause rapid digestion, thus taking away the added fiber benefit. This is why you will find that some whole-grain breads, "brown" breads, pasta and rice, despite looking less refined and being higher in fiber, have a very similar GL to their white counterparts.

Whole grains, flaxseeds and oat fiber are all good sources of insoluble fiber.

Soluble fiber is a gummy mass when mixed with water, and binds with fatty acids which can help lower total and LDL ("bad") cholesterol, reducing the risk of heart disease. It also prolongs stomach-emptying and therefore your feeling of fullness. From the GL stand-point, it slows the release and absorption of sugars into the body and therefore helps regulate blood sugar levels.

Soluble fiber is found in whole oat products and oat bran, legumes, flaxseed, fruits, vegetables and psyllium husk.

Do add extra fiber to your meals and recipes wherever possible, to harness its many benefits—and don't forget to keep hydrated to help the fiber do its job.

Adding Fat and Protein

Adding fat to a food can lower its GL, as it can slow the rate of stomach-emptying and therefore the speed at which a food is digested.

However, this *isn't* a license to add butter to everything!

A good rule is to try and ensure you have a combination of healthy fats, proteins and carbs on your plate. The fats and proteins will help to moderate the effects of the sugars in the carbs, so that overall you should have a lowish GL effect.

Different Types of Foods

Not all foods within the same family will have the same GL. Different types of potatoes, rice and oats have varying GLs, for instance, as they contain different starches which affect the level of starch gelatinization that takes place, and consequently the GL. Not all foods have been tested yet for their GL. We give you the basics in this book, but if you want more specific and up-to-date low-GL food lists, see www.dietfreedom.co.uk.

Chapter 3

HEALTHFUL OILS AND FORGET-ME-NOT FATS

OK, so some fats are GOOD—despite our 20-year indoctrination that ALL FAT is the devil's work, we have finally cleared that one up once and for all (or at least the latest research has).

Virtually ALL dieticians, health professionals and researchers worldwide nowadays agree—it is the *type* of fat you eat that counts, not just the overall quantity.

Fat is essential in our diet, and the majority of it should come from natural oils from **seeds, nuts, olives** and **fish**. These healthful oils are anti-inflammatory, help protect us against heart disease, improve the condition of our nails, hair and skin, can ease depression, and may even help fight cancer.

Types of Fat

Unsaturated Fats—Eat and Enjoy a Good Variety

Monounsaturated—olive oil, avocados, nuts and seeds
Polyunsaturated—seeds, nuts and their oils, oily fish such
   as mackerel, tuna and salmon

Saturated Fats—Eat in Moderation

Found in butter, hard cheeses, coconut oil and fatty
meats

Trans Fats—Avoid!

Hydrogenated margarines are made by converting
vegetable oil into fat at very high temperatures, to make
them last longer. Check labels and avoid anything
containing trans/hydrogenated fats, as they have been
linked with heart disease and cancer. You will find them
in many commercially-produced baked products and in
processed foods, although countries around the world
are now legislating to restrict or ban their use.

What are Essential Fatty Acids (EFAs)?

Fatty acids are the basic building-blocks of all fats and oils. Some of these can be made by the body. The ones the body can't make have to be obtained through the food we eat, and are called **Essential Fatty Acids (EFAs)**. They are "essential" because without them we would die!

EFAs affect our mood, behavior, intelligence and emotions, and are vital to the functioning of the immune system. A lack of them has been linked to depression, chronic fatigue syndrome and, in children, ADHD (Attention Deficit Hyperactivity Disorder), dyslexia and dysphasia.

Signs of deficiency include dry skin, cracked heels, brittle nails, hyperactivity, joint problems, hair loss, dry eyes and digestive disorders.

Good Sources of EFAs

Foods that are rich in EFAs are fish, nuts, seeds, beans, and vegetable oils.

What are Omega 3, 6 and 9?

Essential fatty acids are polyunsaturated and split into two groups—Omega 3 and Omega 6.

We need both Omega 3 and Omega 6 in our diet, but

achieving the right balance of these is not always easy. Many scientists believe that an imbalance of these fatty acids is a major reason for the high incidence of heart disease, diabetes and even some forms of cancer.

Our ancestors evolved on a diet with a ratio of about 1:1, but dramatic changes in our diet mean that today's typical diet provides a ratio closer to 24:1 in favor of Omega 6.

The perfect ratio of these oils is believed to be nearer 5:1 in favor of Omega 6. Most people get enough Omega 6, but it is more difficult to get enough Omega 3 from a modern diet.

Omega 3

The essential Omega 3 fatty acid, ALA, is crucial for brain and eye development, helps prevent abnormal heart rhythms, is important for the immune system and reduces blood-clotting. Two other common Omega 3s are EPA and DHA.

Fish and fish oils are probably the best sources of EPA and DHA, but the content varies depending on the species of fish. The best fish sources are salmon, herring, fresh tuna, pilchards, mackerel and sardines.

All dark green leafy vegetables contain Omega 3, as do some plant-derived oils such as pumpkin seed oil, flaxseed oil and walnut oil.

Omega 6

Omega 6 lowers total blood cholesterol levels as well as "bad" cholesterol (LDL) and is found in cereals, eggs, poultry, whole grain breads and oils such as sunflower, corn, soy and evening primrose.

Omega 9

Omega 9 is not an essential fatty acid, because humans can make it in limited amounts. It is found in almost all natural fats. Avocados, macadamia nuts, apricot seeds, almonds and olive oil are good sources. Omega 9 helps to prevent cancer and boosts the immune system.

Cooking with Oils and Fats

Cooking at high temperatures can damage oils. The more Omega 3 an oil contains, the less suitable it is for cooking. The heat not only damages the fatty acids, it can also change them into harmful substances. The oils that are higher in saturated fats or monounsaturates are the most stable when heated. Best cooking oils and fats are butter (in small amounts), olive oil–based spreads, olive oil, and peanut oil. The main thing to remember when it comes to heating any oils is never to reheat them, as this is when the maximum damage is done.

To preserve the nutritious properties and the flavor of oils you might like to try the "wet-sauté" method practiced by some chefs. Add a couple of tablespoons of water to the pan, heat just below boiling, add the food and cook it lightly before adding the oil, stirring frequently. This shortens the time the oil is in contact with the hot pan. Never heat oils to smoking point, as this damages the fatty acid content and affects the taste adversely. You can still use the more fragile oils at room temperature for dressings.

Storing

Dark bottles are best, as clear glass or plastic bottles allow light to penetrate the oil and oxidize the fatty acids in a chemical process similar to rusting. Store in a cool, dark place and keep the lid on tightly between uses, as contact with air will affect the quality of the oil. Purchase in small quantities and use within a month or two if possible. The healthier the oil, the shorter its shelf-life. Unrefined oils spoil more easily when exposed to warm temperatures, so they need to be refrigerated if you are not going to use them straight away. An exception is olive oil.

Organic

It's definitely worthwhile paying extra for organic oils. Many oils come from plants that are sprayed with pesticides, which are usually fat-soluble, and thus concentrate in the oil portion of the plant. One of the safest oils is extra virgin olive oil, which is not refined or deodorized.

Try and incorporate a variety of oils into your diet, but remember they contain on average 120 calories per tablespoon, so use sparingly. All fats and oils have no GL score as the carb count is negligible.

Avocado oil

History: Avocado seeds were found buried with a mummy dating back to the 8th century BC.

Health bite: Use extra-virgin, cold-pressed. Contains vitamin E and Omega 9.

Everyday uses: Salads or use instead of butter with mashed vegetables.

Coconut oil

History: Coconut oils were recognized as "health oils" in Ayurvedic medicine as far back as 4,000 years ago.

Health bite: Look for virgin coconut oil. Rich in lauric acid, antiviral, antibacterial and antifungal. A saturated fat, so less likely to be damaged when heated.

Everyday uses: Cooking at high temperatures. Very long shelf-life at room temperature.

Flaxseed oil

History: Flaxseed is an ancient grain. Hippocrates wrote of using flax for relief of stomach pains in 650 BC.

Health bite: Rich source of Omega 3 and excellent source of protein, potassium and beta carotene. May help constipation and IBS.

Everyday uses: Delicate nutty flavor, add lemon juice or vinegar for dressings. Keep refrigerated. Short shelf-life. Not suitable for cooking.

Hazelnut oil

History: The word hazel comes from the anglo saxon word *haesel* meaning "bonnet," referring to the shape of the outer shell. Hazelnuts have been cultivated in China for the last 5,000 years.

Health bite: Rich in Vitamin E.

Everyday uses: Nutty, rich and flavorful. A little goes a long way. Use in salad dressings with a bit of olive oil, goes well with asparagus. Can be used in baked goods.

Olive oil

History: The olive dates back to 17th century BC and was mentioned in Egyptian records and several times in the Bible. It has been a sign of peace and truce for millennia.

Health bite: Heart healthy. Doesn't need high temperature or chemical processing, since it is made from the flesh of the olive and not the seed. Look for extra-virgin olive oil as it comes from the first pressing of the olives and is therefore the highest quality.

Everyday uses: Any salad dressings; try mixing with balsamic or red wine vinegar. You can cook with extra-virgin although it is more expensive. Fine for medium-temperature cooking but don't overheat. Good shelf-life.

Peanut oil

History: The peanut originated in Brazil. In 1890 in America it was promoted as a replacement for the cotton crop destroyed by the boll weevil.

Health bite: Contains high levels of plant sterols which research shows may protect against colon, breast and prostate cancer.

Everyday uses: Cooking—especially stir-fries. Has a neutral taste and high burn point.

Pumpkin seed oil

History: First recorded reference in Austria, 1739. Gourmets have appreciated the culinary and health properties of this delicacy for centuries.

Health bite: Healthy monounsaturated fat, helps increase HDL (good cholesterol) and high in zinc.

Everyday uses: Adding flavor to soups, salad dressings. Try mixing with olive oil, mustard and apple vinegar.

Rice bran oil

History: A newcomer on the block. Production first started in the U.S. in the 1960s.

Health bite: A good healthy alternative oil. Great source of vitamin E, antioxidants and micronutrients. Studies in the 1990s have demonstrated it helps reduce cholesterol levels.

Everyday uses: Salads. Also has a very high smoke point, so ideal for pan- and stir-frying. Foods cooked in rice bran oil absorb less oil during cooking. Excellent shelf-life.

Sesame oil

History: Babylonians used it for making exotic perfumes, cooking, sesame cakes and as a medicine. A purchase of sesame oil was recorded on an Egyptian clay tablet in King Nebuchadnezzar's palace records in 6th century BC.

Health bite: High in vitamin E. Dark in color with strong, distinctive flavor.

Everyday uses: Add small amount to stir-fries at end of cooking time, use in salad dressings, or drizzle over steak. Not suitable for cooking. Long shelf-life.

Walnut oil

History: Around 2,000 BC, clay tablets in Mesopotamia revealed the existence of walnut groves within the Hanging Gardens of Babylon. Produced in France, where it is well loved and used widely.

Health bite: Very high in Omega 3.

Everyday uses: Salad dressings: combine it with olive oil. Goes well with fruit, cheese and walnuts, often used with fish. Not suitable for cooking. Short shelf-life.

Flavored/Infused Olive Oils

- **Chili** olive oil—great with mozzarella cheese, tomato sauces or chocolate
- **Garlic** olive oil—good for sauces, pasta, vegetables, fish or meat
- **Basil** olive oil—goes well with rice and pasta salads, soups and tomato sauces
- **Rosemary** olive oil—use with potatoes, fish, beans, risotto or chocolate
- **Lemon** olive oil—ideal for mayonnaise or with white or red meat or tomatoes
- **Ginger** olive oil—good for soups, fish, meat, rice and cakes
- **Porcini mushroom** olive oil—use in risottos, sauces, soups and with vegetables

Chapter 4

GROOVY GRAINS AND FRIENDLY FLOURS

What Are Whole Grains?

When grains are milled or refined, the bran (the fiber-rich outer layer of the kernel) and germ (the nutrient-rich inner part) are removed, leaving only the endosperm (the middle starchy bit). Most of the nutritional value of the grain is lost in the process, because the bran and the germ contain the highest concentration of nutrients.

To increase your intake of whole grains:

- Eat oatmeal which is made from whole-grain oats instead of highly refined cereals. Oats, in general, are a great food choice.
- Swap white bread for whole grain rye/pumpernickel or soy and flaxseed bread.
- Try eating tabbouleh, a popular dish made with bulgur wheat.
- Use pearl barley (great as a rice substitute, as rice is a high-GL food).

- Substitute white flour with flours that are less processed and contain more fiber, such as buckwheat flour, spelt flour, soy flour or gram flour.

When looking at food labels, look for the word "whole" in front of the name of the grain, for example 100 percent whole wheat. Even popcorn is classed as a whole grain!

Eating healthy whole grains fits in very well with your new low-GL eating plan, as whole grains have a lower GL than their highly processed counterparts.

Why Eat Them?

Recent research shows that eating whole grains can help maintain the health of your heart. You will get more benefits from eating whole grains as it is the combination of all three parts of the grain that provide the best health benefits.

Which Whole Grains Are Low GL?

- Bulgur
- Buckwheat
- Corn on the cob and unsweetened popcorn
- Oats (oatmeal makes a great breakfast!)
- Pearl barley

- Quinoa
- Rice generally has a high GL, but wild rice and brown rice tend to have a lower GL than most other varieties—use sparingly or mix half-and-half with pearl barley, quinoa, or beans until you reach your target weight.
- Rye
- Spelt—this is an ancient relative of wheat, and anecdotally (not clinically proven) may be better tolerated than wheat by those with a wheat intolerance. Whole-grain spelt flour has a higher protein and fiber content than most wheat flours, and breads containing spelt have been tested as having a low to moderate GL.
- Wheat—30g of whole wheat has a low GL of 8.
- Gram flour (chickpea flour)—chickpeas have a very low GL, so gram flour and foods containing it should have a lowish GL too.

Why We Can't Test Flours for Their GL

Glycemic testing involves volunteers eating an amount of a specific food that contains 50 grams of carbohydrates, three times! Eating that amount of flour is neither palatable nor advisable and, as you can imagine, volunteers are in short supply!

This is why we can only test foods containing specific flours (such as bread containing spelt flour), which will give us the GL of a portion of spelt flour bread.

Combining Flours—How to Get the Right Mix

It's the gluten in wheat flour that makes bread rise, and as many of the alternative flours don't contain as much gluten, they produce a denser, heavier loaf, which is a good thing GL-wise, as light and fluffy tends to equal quickly digested and therefore high GL.

By using alternative flours such as rye, spelt and buckwheat in a mixture with stoneground 100 percent wholemeal wheat flour, you can create delicious bread variations, a little different in taste and texture from sliced white. Actually they taste far better!

Oats are another great addition to try in the form of oat bran or oatmeal, which give bread a lovely texture. We've also used oatmeal with great success as a crunchy crumb coating for fish and meat.

A generous handful of seeds such as flaxseeds, sunflower seeds or pumpkin seeds in your bread adds to the flavor and will also help lower the GL.

Sourdough breads have a low GL in general, which is thought to be due to the acidic nature of the bread.

Buckwheat flour makes great pancakes—you'll find a recipe on page 110.

Nut flours are very handy in baking, but not much good in bread. They are not as "sticky" as normal flour (because they have no gluten) and you will find that the finished result will be a little more delicate, yet very tasty! Don't forget that nuts are high in calories, and you shouldn't be eating any more than a small handful a day.

Remember that the more refined and processed a flour is, the higher the GL. The coarser the flour, and the more intact it is (i.e. it has not had all its nutritious parts refined away), the better it will be for you not only in terms of having a lower GL but also with regard to its nutritional content. That is why "stoneground" wholemeal flour is better than "brown" or simply "wholemeal" flour. By using the stoneground method of processing, the grains stay more intact.

Thickening

In reality, a spoonful of refined corn starch or plain flour here and there wouldn't be too bad if you don't have anything else, but we have banished them from our kitchens and here is what we use in their place!

- Arrowroot—this is available in the baking section of most grocery stores. It's a ground root, as the name suggests, and is great for thickening. There are instructions on the packet, but in general you just use it the same way you would corn starch (mixing with cold water to a smooth paste before adding to anything). As it has no taste or color, this is our thickener of choice for pretty much all sweet and savory applications.
- Gram flour (chana dal, besan or chickpea flour)—this is made from chickpeas and is a very popular ingredient in Indian cuisine. It makes a good savory

flour and thickener.

- Xanthan gum—this is an effective thickener although a bit fiddly. It needs a lot of whisking as per the packet instructions and does go lumpy very, very quickly! It's not as easy to find or use as arrowroot.
- Buckwheat flour is a reasonable thickener, however don't use in delicately flavored foods as it has a stronger taste and so won't work with everything.
- You can replace high-GL white flours with stoneground 100 percent wholemeal flour in most recipes.
- Spelt flour is also a good thickener. Used exactly as normal white flour, it's great for soufflés and cheese sauces.
- Organic stock cubes and bouillon powder such as the Marigold and Kallo brands make great gravies, but we love them as warming savory drinks too! Make sure you choose organic versions, as non-organic often have hydrogenated fats in them. You can also find low-salt varieties.

A Gluten-free Diet?

What is low-GL AND gluten-free? This is a bit tricky, as many gluten-free products do have a lot of high-GL ingredients and are heavily refined.

Gluten-free corn pastas are generally high-GL, so best avoided. However there are some lovely buckwheat (which is actually part of the rhubarb family!) and chickpea pastas available now (see our website for retailers).

Chickpea flour is a wonderful gluten-free alternative for savory dishes. It works well as a binder and thickener with strong savory flavors.

Spelt flour does contain a small amount of gluten.

Soy flour can be used as a gluten-free flour substitute, however it does have a strong taste that is not palatable to everyone.

Being allergic to wheat is not the same as being allergic to gluten, and so you may be able to eat rye, barley, spelt and oats if it is only wheat that causes you problems.

If you have ANY food allergies or medical conditions, you need to check with your doctor *before* you make any significant changes to your diet. Take this book with you and ask his or her advice before you start.

Chapter 5

HOT HERBS AND SEXY SPICES

We don't add any salt to our recipes, as we all tend to consume far too much as it is. You will find black pepper and other fragrant herbs and spices in the recipes in this book, though, added for their taste, aroma and also, in some cases, their claimed health benefits.

As we are all different in our likes and dislikes, the herbs and spices are very much optional, so don't be put off a recipe if it has a herb or spice that you don't like—just leave it out or add a different one!

There are no hard-and-fast rules as far as we are concerned as to which herb or spice has to "be seen" with a certain food. Experiment—you may be as surprised as we are what combos work really well and become future favorite dishes.

Before we start with the recipes, we thought you might like a list of the most popular, easy-to-find herbs and spices, with some traditional uses plus some fresh ideas and combinations for you to try out. We also love a bit of history, and couldn't resist adding bits here and there with some quaint little anecdotes.

The health properties of herbs and spices are not to be dismissed. Though many of these are anecdotal and not clinically proven, centuries of medics and cooks cannot be ignored!

Top 10 Herbs

Herbs are wonderful things, with amazing properties and a pretty racy past! Doctors, druids, wise women and chefs have been using these plants for centuries to heal, cleanse, repair, boost and flavor.

You don't have to be a green-fingered gardener to enjoy herbs—you can buy them in pots and pluck with impunity, or grow them from seed yourself. Tina likes to buy them in bunches and freeze them, which works really well, and Deborah likes to grow them on the kitchen windowsill and talk to them as she cooks! And we all love the trusty dried herbs in handy shakers.

You can also now buy herbs and spices in convenient tubes and jars, some of which are great, though some do have added sugar and other additives, so always read the label (and see our website for retailers).

Basil

Fresh is best.
Easy to find.
Doesn't freeze well.
Dried is OK.

History: Originally from India, where it is regarded as sacred to the Hindus; also widely used in ancient Rome, Greece and Egypt.

Health bite: A digestive aid, and also a tonic (just the smell will pep you up!). Also used as a stimulant to aid concentration and help combat weariness.

Traditional uses: Basil was taken as a tea to aid digestion, and for a time the dried leaves were made into snuff to combat headaches and colds! Much used in Italian cooking, it goes beautifully with tomatoes, and if you're into growing your own these make great growing partners too.

A new twist: All variations of basil (sweet, purple, lemon, etc.) are delicious and augment any dish, from salads to our own "barleyotto" recipe (page 190). Tear them and add to vegetables and olive oil before roasting. Basil has a delicious flavor and is one of our favorite leaves.

Chives

Fresh is best.
Dried is OK.
Freezes well in water in ice cube trays.

History: Chives have been cultivated for over 5,000 years, and are thought to have originated in China.

Health bite: Chives are reputed as a general tonic.

Traditional uses: Chives have always been associated with egg dishes, cream cheese, fish and chicken.

A new twist: Add at the last minute to literally anything! A liberal sprinkling of fresh chives and a squeeze of lemon juice gives incredible zing to almost any dish we can think of, particularly steamed veggies.

Cilantro

Fresh is best for the leaves.
Seeds are dried—best to crush them as and when needed.

History: Aphrodisiac! It has long been reputed to aid *amour*, and was also used in parts of Arabia to ease labor pains and regulate the reproductive system.

Health bite: The essential oil is used to combat poor circulation, digestive problems and colds/flu. Cilantro seed tea is used to aid digestion.

Traditional uses: Most used in China, Thailand, Mexico, the southern Mediterranean and the Middle East. Often added to curries, pickles and breads.

A new twist: Stir the leaves through couscous or bulgur wheat, sprinkle on grilled halloumi, use instead of basil to make a pesto, add as a leaf to salads for extra zing. Crush the seeds, and warm in a pan, pour over 1 tbsp of olive oil and use as a warm dressing for halloumi cheese.

Fennel

Fresh is best.
The seeds are dried and can be crushed or added whole.

History: A Mediterranean native, it was brought to Northern Europe by the Romans. One of the 9 sacred herbs of the Anglo Saxons, it is surrounded by much myth and is a favorite of the "white witch."

It has a reputation for helping eyesight, and was also mixed with straw in kennels and stables to keep away fleas!

Health bite: It is still used by some herbalists to relieve dry tired eyes, earache, toothache, asthma, coughs (it's in many cough mixtures, and gripe water) and rheumatism. It is also a digestive aid and mild laxative.

Traditional uses: The seeds were used in pasta, bread and biscuits to help with the digestion of these starchy foods. The leaves were traditionally laid as a bed upon which to bake a whole fish, gently infusing it with the slight aniseed flavor.

A new twist: Braise the chopped bulbs in white wine for a lovely side dish, or use in place of onion in stir-frys and roasted vegetable combos. Drink the tea made from infusing the seeds as a digestive aid instead of coffee after a meal. Add the finely chopped leaves—only a teaspoon or so—to salads. Fennel is particularly good with oily fish.

Garlic

Fresh is best.
Smoked garlic is wonderful!
Tubes and jars are great but check for added sugar or nasties.
Dried is a good store cupboard standby.

History: Garlic was much used by the Romans, who would chew on raw garlic before battle! Its properties have been lauded by famous literati, including Shakespeare, Chaucer and Pliny. It has been acknowledged for centuries as a plant with great health benefits.

Health bite: Garlic is a natural antiseptic and has blood-cleansing properties. It helps battle colds and flu and boosts the immune system.

Traditional uses: As an intestinal "cleanse," to lower blood pressure, get rid of worms, alleviate chest infections, and help with the symptoms of rheumatism. In the First World War, the raw juice was used on wounds as an effective antiseptic.

A new twist: Roast whole cloves in their skin (or an entire head!) with your next roast, and then squeeze out the sweet cooked garlic—it is truly a magical flavor. Infuse a bottle of olive oil with garlic by peeling and slicing the garlic into the bottle. Use a few drops of this with some lemon juice as a salad zinger or as a great pre-cook marinade for chicken or fish.

Thyme

Fresh is best.
Freezes well.
Freeze loose in bags and you'll find the leaves will easily shake
from the stalks, making it very convenient.
Dried works well too.

History: Another Mediterranean native, thyme absorbs the sun better than most other plants and is packed with medicinal qualities. Has been traditionally used for centuries in pies, stuffings, stews and patés.

Health bite: Thyme has been used for the treatment of colds, coughs, colic and cramps. It is also a digestive and appetite stimulant. An infusion makes a good mouthwash.

Traditional uses: Garden thyme is most traditionally used in the "mixed herbs" blend (with sage and marjoram) and also in "bouquet garni" with parsley, marjoram and bay. Garden and lemon thyme are the two most often used in the kitchen, though there are many ornamental varieties that look wonderful and smell incredible in the garden.

A new twist: It makes a great bed on which to bake chicken pieces, and augments tomato-based sauces very well. Add the fresh leaves to salads, sparingly, or mix in with the dressing. You can infuse a light wine vinegar with lemon thyme for a wonderfully fragrant salad dressing.

Parsley

Fresh is best.
Easy to find.
Freezes well.
Dried doesn't work very well.

History: In Greek mythology, parsley sprung from the blood of the hero Archemorous, the forerunner of death—so it was important in their burial rituals. Warriors fed their chariot horses parsley. It is thought to originate in Sardinia. Old wives have it that it thrives only in the gardens of dominant women!

Health bite: The foliage of both the flat and curly parsley is packed with vitamins A, B, and C and iron. Parsley tea is given to aid circulation and digestion and to assist the kidneys.

Traditional uses: All parts of the plant are useful, with the roots and larger stems being traditionally blanched and eaten as vegetables. The seeds have also been used in the making of cheese—though the seeds are rarely used now. Parsley stalks are often included in "bouquet garni."

A new twist: Add to salads in abundance with other leaves and herbs for a vitamin-packed and tasty alternative. It is a fresh-tasting and mild herb, so can be used for color in almost any leafy setting. Add fresh, finely chopped leaves to mashed veggies.

Mint

Fresh is best.
Easy to find.
Easy to grow.
Freezes well.

History: Stories of mint date back to Greek mythology and biblical times, when it was strewn liberally on floors for its sweet cooling scent and insect-repelling properties as well as being used to scent bath water. In Saxon Britain it was known as "the monk's herb" as it was so well used by them.

Health bite: Peppermint, spearmint and lemon mint all make a very refreshing and uplifting tea. It is a digestive and may help calm the stomach after meals or when feeling delicate. It will help unblock the sinuses, and is renowned as a natural aid to a deep, restful sleep. It is also said to have a beneficial cumulative effect in building up a resistance to colds.

Traditional uses: All varieties of mint were reputed to stop milk from curdling. Leaves of the "eau de cologne" mint were added to the bath for a cooling experience. It is also used in Benedictine, crème de menthe and Chartreuse.

A new twist: In the summer make iced peppermint tea—pour hot water over fresh mint and let steep for a while, then top up with cold water, strain, add ice cubes and fresh mint leaves and refrigerate. Use mint generously in salads and with freshly steamed veggies. Mint and freshly squeezed pomegranate juice makes a great salad dressing. Try tossing watermelon and feta cheese chunks with lots of torn fresh mint leaves, some lemon juice and a little olive oil.

Rosemary

Fresh is best.
Easy to find.
Easy to grow.
Freezes well in a bag, coming easily off the stalk when you need it.
Dried is a good standby.

History: Considered a magic and sacred herb in many cultures.

Greek students used to weave rosemary in their hair in ancient times while studying for exams. It has also long been used as a natural insect repellent.

Health bite: Rosemary is used in hair tonics and anti-dandruff shampoos to stimulate the scalp, encouraging shiny, healthy hair. It is used as a herbal cure for "nervous" headaches. It has a "bracing" aroma and is great added to your bath in the morning to aid consciousness!

Traditional uses: Oil of rosemary was used in the original "eau de cologne." Rosemary is also a traditional plant of remembrance, used in Australia on Anzac (Remembrance) Day as a buttonhole. Traditionally it is used with lamb and heavy meats, however while it is a strong herb, it's a lot more versatile than that, so don't be afraid to experiment!

A new twist: Add 2 tablespoons of fresh chopped leaves to any low-GL bread recipe for a lovely pungent lift to your morning toast! Add some freshly chopped rosemary to any pasta or bean dish, particularly if using tomatoes. It goes very well with steamed cabbage—put a sprig of fresh rosemary into the steamer first, then steam the cabbage on top of it. Wash the leaves and dry carefully—add to olive oil or light vinegar for a wonderful dressing/marinade standby.

Sage

Fresh is best.
Freezes very well.
Dried is a good standby.

History: Sage is another Mediterranean native, reputed to be one of the magic ingredients for eternal life! Was used by the Egyptians to boost their intellectual powers and revive a tired brain after much exertion.

Health bite: Reputed to aid memory and help boost energy levels. It is a very well-known antiseptic ingredient used in mouthwashes. Can also help alleviate indigestion and heartburn. Sage tea can be taken as a tonic for the liver and the nerves.

Traditional uses: Sage has been used in tea, cheeses, breads and hair tonics (apparently stops you from going gray!) for centuries. It was also traditionally used with pork, duck and goose. It works well in cheese dishes, and is used in cheese production.

A new twist: If you're feeling sluggish, have a cup of sage tea in the morning—made with fresh or dry leaves. A sprinkling of finely chopped sage in any salad is lovely. It goes very well with fresh tuna or other oily fish—sprinkle fresh chopped leaves over the top, or incorporate dried sage into a dressing. It also goes well with eggs, cheese, and tomatoes and gives a lift to vegetable soups (especially pea soup). A generous handful inside a roast chicken imparts a lovely flavor.

Top 10 Spices

The fate of countries and dynasties have risen and fallen with spices. Use of spices can be traced as far back as 3500 BC to the ancient Egyptians, who used them not only in food but also in cosmetics and for embalming their dead.

King Solomon's vast wealth was attributed to spices. The Chinese were very enterprising spice-traders, dealing with Arab traders who went to great pains not to pass on their jealously guarded spice routes to their customers.

While the dominant trading power in the Mediterranean changed from Egypt to Babylon and then Assyria, the Arabs held on to their role as the suppliers of these exotic wares for many years. Incredible stories were told by these canny traders about snake-infested pits of cinnamon and mythical, vicious winged birds that guarded various spice crops.

It was the Romans who introduced spices into Northern Europe.

The religious Crusades started the spice wars, and spices were, for a time, more precious than gold and silver due to their rarity.

Marco Polo was first to dispel the myths about fearsome beasts guarding the spices. His book, written while in prison, inspired future generations of spice traders.

The year 1400 AD brought the so-called Age of Discovery and a Europe-wide obsession with finding the best spice route to the East. Vasco da Gama from Portugal was the first round the Cape of Good Hope, coming home to Lisbon with trade agreements and a ship laden with spices. Christopher Columbus found the New World, bringing home chilies, allspice and vanilla as well as chocolate, maize and peanuts. Magellan and Drake both made their names—and incredible discoveries—in the name of spice!

The Dutch and British soon took over, and their bloody battle for spice supremacy lasted nearly 200 years.

Today we take these readily available exotic ingredients for granted, and it is very hard for us to imagine a time when a handful of cardamom was worth more than some people's annual wage!

Next time you use a spice, it's worth remembering that the fate of nations and many lives have hung in the balance over them—their taste and aromas have launched many ships and sparked huge exploration, and they have, in fact, played a major part in the shape of the world as we know it today.

Allspice

The best flavor comes from the whole seeds ground as you need them.

History: Allspice is the berry of a tree native to the West Indies and Central America. It is also known as Jamaica pepper or pimento. The dried berries of this type of myrtle tree are very hard and smell of a combination of cinnamon, nutmeg and cloves.

Health bite: The essential oil of the berries and leaves are used in preparations for flatulence and are also antiseptics.

Traditional uses: Allspice is almost always ground, and was traditionally used in mulled wines, fruit cakes, fruit and steamed puddings and is an integral part of many spice blends. Many Scandinavian and German dishes use allspice.

A new twist: Add ½ teaspoon of ground allspice to mashed squash or sweet potatoes, or mix into some olive oil and drizzle over before you bake these veggies. Put a teaspoon in with a meatball mix, or in with a winter stew. Add a teaspoon to some fine oatmeal, along with some black pepper, mix well and use as a crispy coating for fried herring.

Chili

There are so many types of chilies it's hard to say which are best—choose your favorites, fresh or dried, and approach any unknown chilies with caution!
If you've got a greenhouse or conservatory you can easily grow your own.

History: The chili is an American native, and there are many different types, strengths and flavors. The Aztecs used to blend cocoa and chili for a pungent and spicy hot chocolate very far removed from the modern-day version!

Health bite: While chilies are rich in vitamin C, you are unlikely to eat enough to make a health difference. Chilies do stimulate the appetite and cool down the body, particularly in the hotter climates. If you eat too hot a chili, yogurt or milk are the best ways to cool down your mouth quickly.

Traditional uses: Hot dishes, curries, Thai and Mexican cuisine all rely on various types of chilies, from the searingly hot bird's-eye chilies to the slightly milder cayenne version. Many milder chilies are dried and smoked and add wonderful warmth and flavor to stews, marinades and sauces.

A new twist: If you get the chance to test different chili powders or fresh chilies, then do. They can add wonderful depth and pungency to a dish, not just heat. Add a pinch to steamed cabbage, toss with a little olive oil and some garlic for a really fresh side dish. Add a pinch of smoky passilia chilies to a tablespoon of half-fat cream cheese or hummus for a delicious dip.

Cinnamon

It's more pungent if bought in sticks and ground as needed, however it is very handy ready-ground and still tastes great.

History: This exotic spice is made from the ground bark of a tree native to Ceylon (Sri Lanka) and Malabar. It has been much sought-after since biblical times, when it was valued above gold. Cinnamon is an ancient herbal medicine mentioned in Chinese texts as long as 4,000 years ago.

Health bite: Has a broad range of historical uses in different cultures. Believed to be helpful for diabetes, colic, indigestion, heartburn and yeast infections. Test-tube studies show that cinnamon can augment the action of insulin. However, use of cinnamon to improve the action of insulin for diabetics has not been proven in clinical trials.

Traditional uses: Mulled wines, stewed fruits, cakes, puddings and biscuits and, more recently, sprinkled on coffee in coffee bars.

A new twist: A teaspoon of cinnamon in your oatmeal in the morning will give it a real lift. Include cinnamon instead of sugar in your coffee, or use a cinnamon stick as your coffee stirrer for an aromatic brew. Put a pinch in winter stews for wonderful warmth.

Cardamom

Best bought in pods and split/crushed as needed.

History: Cardamom bushes reputedly grew in the Hanging Gardens of Babylon.

Health bite: Cardamom cools the body and aids digestion. It has been used for millennia as a tooth-whitener and breath-freshener. It is used in Ayurvedic medicine as a cure for urinary tract and skin complaints.

Traditional uses: Indian curries, sweetmeats and ice cream all employ cardamom, and it's used a great deal in Scandinavian cooking. Arabian coffee is often brewed with or poured through cardamoms.

A new twist: Include a sprinkling of cardamom pods in the gravy for any roast meat. Split the pods, crush the seeds and sprinkle in with beans, rice, our own "barley-otto" recipe (page 190). Also adds an extra dimension to stir-fries.

Cumin

Best bought as seeds and "dry fried" for about 30 seconds before adding to anything, or crushed, which improves the flavor.

History: Cumin comes from Egypt and has been found in the pyramids. It has been grown for centuries in the Mediterranean, the Middle East and India, is mentioned in the Bible, and was very popular in the UK in the Middle Ages.

Health bite: Widely reputed to be good for the stomach. Also much used in veterinary medicines, and the oil is used in perfumes.

Traditional uses: One sniff will tell you it is another traditional ingredient in curry powder. It is also used in Moroccan and Mexican cooking.

A new twist: Cut one pack of halloumi cheese into thin slices, toast a teaspoon of cumin seeds in a hot pan, add 1 tablespoon olive oil and then fry the halloumi until golden. Add to stews, or crush and mix with olive oil and brush on meat before grilling.

Ginger

Fresh is definitely best, and it freezes in chunks (don't bother to peel) making it very quick and easy to grate and always have on standby. Dried ginger has a deeper, warmer flavor and is used in sweet baking.

History: Ginger is king of the spices in our book! Its first mention on the page appears to be in the writings of the Eastern philosopher Confucius in 500 BC. Henry VIII was a fan, and the renowned herbalist Culpepper also sang its praises.

Health bite: Renowned for anti-nausea properties, and great for the digestive system. Also aids absorption, often used in Chinese medicine to speed the absorption of the herbal remedies prescribed. Also known to help reduce fevers and cold symptoms.

Traditional uses: Crystallized and powdered in sweet cakes and biscuits and fresh in Chinese cookery. It is also used widely in Indian cuisine.

A new twist: Add about 1 tsp fresh grated ginger, a pinch of hot chili flakes and a clove of crushed or grated garlic to a pan, add 40g cooked brown rice per person, and a handful of butterbeans. Stir-fry for about 2 minutes, then serve as a delicious spicy side dish to most meats.

Mustard

Seeds, ready-made, powder—choose your favorite and enjoy it! Avoid ready-made mustards that contain flour.

History: White mustard is native to Europe, and black mustard, which is hotter, to Asia and Africa. A mustard paste was recommended by Pythagoras as a treatment for scorpion stings.

Health bite: Mustard baths and footbaths were said to ease all manner of muscular aches. It is reputed to be good for the respiratory system.

Traditional uses: Although mostly grown for the seeds, mustard greens have been eaten in salads or as a spinach alternative for centuries. Ground mustard powder is another staple of many curry blends. It is traditionally served with beef.

A new twist: Add grainy mustard to cauliflower mash. It really complements the flavors of oily fish, mushrooms and cheese. Spread thinly over rye bread and drape with smoked salmon.

Nutmeg

Buy whole and grate as needed to keep the flavor at its most pungent.

History: The popularity of nutmeg hit its zenith in the 17th century, and only started to wane in the 19th century. The tongue-twister "Peter Piper" relates to nutmeg and mace (same fruit) and a Frenchman called Peter Poivre who successfully broke the monopoly the Dutch had taken from the Portuguese in the trading of nutmeg and mace in the 1700s.

Health bite: Reputed to cure flatulence and assist the digestion of rich foods. Nutmeg is an astringent, a stimulant and, apparently, an aphrodisiac.

Traditional uses: Traditionally has been used with eggs, cheese and spinach as well as in sweet products such as biscuits, custards and spicy cakes. It is also one of the ingredients in traditional mulled wines. The oil is also used in perfumes and ointments.

A new twist: Grate over wilted spinach. Grate into mushroom or pumpkin soup. Grate over vegetables before roasting, particularly squash. Grate into your cauliflower mash. Grate into stewed apple. Grate a little into your hot chocolate or coffee.

Paprika

Paprika is most often found powdered.
Smoked paprika is wonderful, too.

History: From the same family as the chili and a native of America. The large, aromatic capsicums are dried and ground. Though grown in many countries, the best quality is said to come from Hungary and is known as "Noble Sweet." Paprika is also known as "Grains of Paradise."

Health bite: Paprika is rich in vitamin C, though there are no other notable health benefits associated with it— so enjoy it just for its wonderful warmth and flavor!

Traditional uses: Hungarian goulash, paprika chicken. It is also very popular in Spanish and Portuguese cooking. It is a very common commercial flavoring and coloring agent.

A new twist: Paprika, through "smoked paprika," is enjoying something of a revival currently, and its warm smoky flavor brings welcome depth to cheese, chicken, egg and fish dishes.

Pepper

Peppercorns in a mill freshly ground as you need them retain far more flavor and pungency than ready-ground pepper.

History: Originally from the East Indies, all color berries come from the same plant. The Romans used it a great deal because it was a relatively cheap spice. Rents in the Middle Ages were often paid in peppercorns due to their high value and scarcity, and the term "peppercorn rent" at that time meant payment in full.

Health bite: It is said to be good for anemia, a sluggish digestion, nausea and stiff joints, and to be a real tonic to help oust colds and flu.

Traditional uses: Traditionally, white pepper was used for white food, black pepper for "coarse" food. It was also used as a meat preservative. Pepper is now the most widely used spice and works well in almost any dish—including some fruit!

A new twist: Freshly ground black pepper for all things! Experiment with fruit, such as strawberries with finely ground pepper; or with figs and goat's cheese.

Chapter 6

LOW-GL SWEETNESS

Yes, we could say banish all sweetness from your life, but we aren't going to for several reasons—(all sweet-lovers punch air at this point)—the first one is that sweet is nice ... and savory, albeit delightful, can be a bit of a bore when it's your only choice.

If you cast your mind back to the low-carb diets, when meat, fish, eggs, cheese and chemical sweeteners or "run to the bathroom" polyols were the order of the day ... what boring days they were.

So you will be pleased to hear that we aren't going to ask you to banish ALL sugars from your diet and replace them with nasty-tasting chemical alternatives, which may or may not have side-effects—the jury still being out on that one. And we certainly don't want to take the risk of replacing one "not great for you" ingredient for another. Besides, we wouldn't advocate anything that we don't eat ourselves or don't believe to be good for you.

So where does that lead us—can we really have sweetness *and* goodness, or are the two mutually exclusive? Well, we have scratched our heads over this one for many a moon—how to find sweetness and goodness with a low GL?

Fruit is a great sweetener—chop it, squeeze it, purée it, liquidize it and generally shake it about; add it to oatmeal, muesli, yogurt, fry it in olive oil and add it to savory dishes—and if it is low-GL fruit (and most of them are), all the lovelier.

At this point you may be thinking how you hate washing the blender, or haven't got one, or have got one in the loft, competing for dust with the cappuccino machine and the ice cream maker ... and that every time you have bought fresh fruit in the past it has been discovered sitting at the back of the fridge with a furry coat on a week later.

Fear not. You can buy puréed fruit now with no added sugar (see our website for retailers) plus you can get some nice fruit juices (some mixed with vegetables) without added sugar, too—so you won't have to do anything except tear off the top and pour—quite painless in fact. So we can all have some sweetness in our lives with good old-fashioned fabulous fruit.

"But," say the clever cooks among us, "we can't bake without sugar ... it's ... it's *unheard* of!" Well, good news: YES YOU CAN and should. The empty calories in sugar aren't the only way we can make things taste and look good. Our current best of the best available now that are sweet AND good are:

Agave syrup—a delicious, natural low-GL sweetener made from the same plant that tequila comes from. It has fewer calories than sugar, is sweeter (so you can use up to a third less), takes less time to cook AND has a low GL. It is much thinner than honey, so is easy to use and "pourable" from a bottle. You can also add it to oatmeal or yogurt, and it mixes easily with cocoa to make a delicious low-GL chocolate syrup/sauce (see page 252 for recipe).

You can now also buy **crystalline fructose**, which has a much lower GL than sugar and, since it's a third sweeter, you can use less. Use on its own or mix with fruit purée to replace sugar in baking.

Don't confuse *"fructose"* with *"high fructose corn syrup,"* which is a high-GL sweetener used by the food industry.

The Lowdown on Polyols (Sugar Alcohols)

These sweeteners are being added to more and more so-called low-carb products by the day, and recently some products claiming to be low GI/GL, but you need to be aware that they are controversial, as are the "net carb" claims used on packaging.

Manufacturers are putting the actual carb count in very small print on the back of the product (polyols are high in carbs) but then claiming that you don't need to count them as carbs—hence the low "net carbs" figure. Their reasoning is that polyols are digested differently than normal carbs and therefore can be discounted; however, this is still a controversial issue, particularly as there are numerous different types of polyols on the market, all with varying effects.

The main issue, however, is that they can cause some very unpleasant side-effects—namely chronic flatulence and emergency visits to the bathroom! If you have irritable bowel syndrome then they are best avoided, as they can seriously aggravate it.

The main polyols used worldwide are:

- xylitol
- erythritol
- HSH (hydrogenated starch hydrolysates)
- isomalt
- lactitol
- maltitol
- mannitol
- sorbitol

Polyols are chemical reductions of starches and sugar molecules, but they are, in fact, neither sugar nor alcohol.

The term can be confusing, as "sugar alcohols" are not digested like sugar, nor do they have the same effect as alcohol.

Polyols are carbohydrates, but their different chemical structures affect how thoroughly we absorb them. Polyols break down slowly and are incompletely absorbed from the small intestine into the blood, because there is no specific transport mechanism in the body for their absorption. Some of the polyols are absorbed and some broken down in the large intestine and metabolized into short-chain fatty acids, which are then absorbed and used for fuel (and which count as calories).

Intestinal bacteria ferment the rest, producing gases which can cause gastrointestinal distress, followed by strange sounds, bloating and sometimes diarrhea. Any undigested part of the polyols is excreted. Products containing polyols must carry a warning—"Excess consumption may have a laxative effect." All polyols have the capacity to produce intestinal discomfort.

As there appear to be differences in the way different polyols are absorbed, we all have a different level of tolerance to them. Some people may experience gastrointestinal discomfort after eating as little as 10 grams—and a single serving of a polyol-sweetened product could include twice that amount. If you eat several foods containing polyols throughout the day, the grams soon stack up and you can end up with a very embarrassing problem!

So, treat foods containing polyols with caution, and bear in mind that although there are different types, consuming too many polyols is likely to cause gastrointestinal distress. (It has also been suggested that consuming polyols can prove fatal to pets, so please be aware.) You may also find that relying on "net carbs" as trumpeted on labels is not a good indicator as to the food's effect on your body or weight-loss efforts.

Many other artificial sweeteners such as aspartame are low-GL, but we will leave it for you to decide whether you want to include them in your diet or not. Personally we avoid them as they aren't natural and are controversial healthwise.

If you want to buy a sweet treat, look for natural products sweetened with a *small* amount of fructose, natural honey or agave syrup, as these should have a lowish glycemic impact without any side-effects.

A great semi-sweet treat is 70%-plus cocoa dark chocolate. Since it contains so much cocoa, there isn't room for much sugar. In addition, cocoa is good for us so it is fine to eat this product in small quantities or to use occassionally in recipes.

Chapter 7

GENERAL GUIDELINES FOR SUCCESS

Swapping High-GL Ingredients for Low Ones

You will find no sugar or white flour in any of our recipes. Both are replaced with lower-GL, less processed and less refined, more natural substitutes. You won't find any added salt, either, and you won't need it! We do, however, like our herbs and spices ... a lot—and use them instead of salt as a great taste-enhancer. They also have lots of health benefits and colorful histories, as you've seen in Chapter 5!

Thankfully the food industry is now taking an interest in producing ingredients that have a low GL, so the choices are ever-expanding. Until recently the major concern was the fat and calorie content of foods, but this is changing rapidly. Now the focus is moving towards ingredients and products that have a low GL, do not contain unhealthy hydrogenated or trans fats, are low in salt, have no added sugars and are as natural and unprocessed as possible. Whole grains are also becoming a health focus as research proves their nutritional and health benefits.

It may take some time, possibly years, until we have low-GL substitutes for all of the high-GL, highly processed ingredients now out there, but we have made sure that the recipes in this book are as natural as possible and that they are all low-GL except for the odd exception as noted.

So you don't need to worry about anything, we have done all the working out for you so you can just follow the recipes—enjoy your scrumptious low-GL meals and lose weight (or just feel better) as a welcome side-effect!

We have also put together a low-GL "swapping list" for you—so you can see at a glance some of the ingredient substitutes you can make. Do experiment to find your favorite mixes.

Your Swapping List

High GL (avoid)	Low GL (try instead)
Sugar (brown and white)	❑ small amount of fructose or agave syrup
See Chapter 6	(see www.dietfreedom.co.uk for retailers)
	Fructose is not the same as high-fructose corn syrup, which is a highly processed, high-GL ingredient to be avoided.
	No more than a dessert spoon of agave OR fructose per day.

High GL (avoid)	Low GL (try instead)
White flour *See Chapter 4*	❑ oat flour ❑ soy flour ❑ nut flours (such as almond, walnut, etc.) ❑ gram flour *(made from chickpeas, does have quite a strong savory taste so you may want to use sparingly or mix with other flours)* ❑ buckwheat flour ❑ spelt flour ❑ stoneground wholemeal flour ❑ quinoa flour *Again, although generally products made with these flours will have a lower GL than products made with highly processed white flours, they are still high in carbohydrates so use only in moderation.*
White bread	❑ darker, denser whole grain bread ❑ soy and flaxseed bread ❑ sourdough bread ❑ pumpernickel/rye bread *Women, no more than 1 slice per day; men, no more than 2 slices per day while in weight-loss mode.*

High GL (avoid)	Low GL (try instead)
Potatoes	❑ new potatoes
	❑ sweet potatoes
	❑ yams
	❑ other vegetables
	❑ beans
	An average portion would be 80g. Don't exceed this amount of potatoes in a day.
	Recent research shows that cooking potatoes and refrigerating them before eating lowers the GL, as does adding a vinegar-based dressing.

High GL (avoid)	Low GL (try instead)
White rice	❏ pearl barley
	❏ buckwheat
	❏ wild rice
	❏ brown rice
	Only eat small portions of rice—no more than a handful—combine with beans
	❏ chickpeas
	❏ butterbeans
	❏ pinto beans
	❏ haricot beans
	❏ cannellini beans
	❏ lentils
	❏ quinoa
	any beans or a "combo" of the above – whichever you have in the cupboard!
Pasta (white)	❏ chickpea pasta
	❏ buckwheat pasta
	❏ mixed beans
	❏ whole wheat pasta *(no more than a handful)*
	vegetable pasta—julienned vegetables, blanched, drained and served with pasta sauce

High GL (avoid)	Low GL (try instead)
Ripe fruit	❏ firm, less ripe fruit—this has a lower GL *The vast majority of fruits are low GL—tropical fruits tend to have a higher GL than others such as berries. The less processed and closest to their original form, the better.* *The fiber in the skin (where edible) helps to slow the rate of digestion and the glycemic response.* *Ripe bananas have a far higher GL than unripe.*
Milk Chocolate	❏ dark chocolate with 70%+ cocoa content and minimal sugar *Combine agave syrup with cocoa to make a delicious, natural, low-GL chocolate sauce—see recipe page 252.*
Corn starch/ wheat flour as thickeners	❏ Arrowroot, which works in the same way as corn starch and is available from almost all grocery stores in the baking section. *Use as per instructions on the packet.*

Food Notes

Milk

Your choice! Choose from cow's, goat's, sheep's or soy milk—you can also use coconut milk, oat milk and nut milk for a change. Up to half a pint a day. You can choose which milk you prefer to use, but bear in mind that the recipes are based on using lowfat cow's milk, so if you use something else the results may vary slightly.

Yogurt

All yogurts without added sugars have a low GL. Choose a natural, sugar-free yogurt, bio-yogurt or Greek yogurt. If you are concerned about your saturated fat intake then use lowfat yogurt versions, just make sure they have no added sugar. The lowfat natural "bio" yogurts are generally more creamy in texture. Aim to eat the equivalent of a small tub of yogurt every day.

Cheese

All cheese is low GL. As per yogurt you can choose lower-fat cheeses such as Edam or ones that state "low or reduced fat" on the packaging. They generally taste really good. If you prefer full-fat cheese, just limit the amount used. Don't eat more than 2.6 oz. of lowfat or 1.8 oz. of high-fat cheese per day.

Herbs

Herbs and spices won't add to your GL. You can use either dried herbs or the puréed herbs in tubes (check they have no sugar or additives) instead of fresh in most recipes, although the results may not be quite as good. Freezing fresh herbs works really well. See Chapter 5 for the low-down on herbs and spices, and remember that if you don't like a herb or spice in a recipe, swap it for something you do—or omit them altogether if you prefer.

Fats

Fat doesn't add to your GL score. In fact, both fat and protein eaten at the same time as carbohydrates help to slow down the speed of digestion and therefore lower your glycemic response to the overall meal.

Use either olive oil or olive oil–based spreads (no trans/hydrogenated fats) for frying and baking. A small amount of butter is fine now and then if you prefer.

Vegetables

Virtually all vegetables have a low GL—so enjoy! An average portion would be around 80g. Just avoid normal white potatoes—try to use new potatoes or sweet potatoes instead. Again, 80g would be a sensible portion, and you should aim for three portions of vegetables per day.

Fruit

Most fresh fruit has a low GL. Ripe bananas are one exception, so just go for a small banana that is yellow-and-green striped instead.

Some dried fruits such as dates, figs, raisins and currants have a high GL, so are best avoided. Go for dried apricots, apple, mango and cranberries instead, but make sure they have no added sugar. One or two portions of fruit a day (alongside your three vegetable portions) is ideal.

Meat and Fish

All meat and fish is carbohydrate-free so won't add to your GL. Follow the healthy eating guidelines in Chapter 1 regarding meat and fish.

Nuts and Seeds

Both are very good for you but very calorie-dense, so limit to a small handful a day if you want to lose weight.

Should We All Buy Organic?

You can follow a low-GL diet by buying "everyday" foods, and many people do just that because the cost of buying organic plus lots of "special" ingredients can mount up. But it has to be said that, for some foods, switching to organic makes a lot of sense.

Organic foods are becoming more and more popular every year as we all become increasingly aware of the food that we eat, where it comes from and, in the case of animals, how they were treated and what they were treated with (i.e. antibiotics and hormones) prior to arriving on our plates. Consumers are becoming more demanding as factory farming and the methods used to fatten animals ever faster and more profitably are now under the media spotlight in a big way.

The food we buy nowadays can come from practically anywhere in the world, so it makes perfect sense to be cautious about what we choose to eat and what we provide for our families.

Many grocery stores are now offering a wider range of organic and cruelty-free foods, so do check them out and, if in doubt—ASK!

If buying all organic is a bit of a financial stretch, at least try to buy organic meats, poultry and organic or free-range eggs.

Organic meat comes from animals that have been raised using more traditional methods, hence the higher cost. If you are concerned about animal cruelty, buy organic. It tastes far better and will be free from antibiotic residues, which is important for our future health. Conventional farmers often add antibiotics to animal food to make animals grow faster, so when we eat the meat we absorb many of the antibiotic residues, which could cause future problems as we are becoming more and more resistant to all sorts of antibiotics. The fewer antibiotics you are exposed to, the fewer you'll be resistant to.

So even if you have to buy smaller portions to keep the cost the same, your body will thank you in the long run!

If you can stretch to organic fruit and vegetables as well, even better, as you will avoid the chemical residues and get more nutrients for your money. Mineral levels of organic fruit and vegetables can be 100 percent higher than non-organic, and they contain less water than those grown using fertilizers and chemical sprays, so you get far more quality and less water for your money. It's a sobering thought that the fruit and vegetables you eat as an individual each year will probably have been sprayed with a gallon of herbicides and pesticides!

You may have noticed that a lot of fruit and vegetables are quite tasteless nowadays. This is due to their high water content. Some tomatoes taste just like water, and the same goes for some apples!

With food, as with most things in life, you get what you pay for—make cutbacks elsewhere, but making the quality of the food you eat your priority is the best thing you can do for your own and your family's health.

The world's top chefs use organic produce in their restaurants for the quality and taste. If you haven't tried organic meat, fish or poultry—try it, you won't go back!

Convenience and Canned Foods

Canned food is a great store cupboard standby. Just check for added sugars and salt. Even canned vegetables such as peas and carrots can have sugar added!

Canned fruit is OK providing it isn't in a sugar-laden syrup. Fresh fruit is obviously better but if you do buy cans look for the ones in their own juice with no sugar added.

Baked beans are probably the most popular canned food, but again, they all have sugar added. You can get cans of organic baked beans sweetened with a small amount of apple juice. See our website for retailers. The same rule applies to any other convenience foods. Check the labels for added sugar and choose organic where possible.

Chapter 8

7-DAY RECIPE SELECTOR

We are all deliciously different!

No two people reading this book are the same, and neither are we, so we have split the recipes up into different sections. Tina is the "fast and friendly" recipe fiend—her criteria being "if it tastes good, looks good, is healthy AND can be thrown together in a few minutes, marvelous and all the more enjoyable!" You won't find any of Tina's recipes taking more than 20 minutes start to finish, as Tina (and we are sure a few of you out there too) has reached her boredom threshold by then!

Deborah, on the other hand, finds cooking a relaxing and soothing thing, a form of therapy even, so she is more than happy to peel and chop and stir and marinate for as long as it takes to get to the end result. Deborah has devised the "foodie-friendly" recipes, so be prepared for a bit of prep work here and a bit more time spent.

Both of us are very keen on vegetables, so we have combined our approaches to create the "veggie-friendly" recipes.

Nigel is kind of in-between depending on his mood and the time he has to spend (not that he is moody, you understand!).

And we'd like to take a minute here to thank Diet Freedom online Club members Andie, Olivia, Lorraine, Selina, Caroline, Sally and Lesley for kindly passing on some lovely recipes to us, which we have included in the chapters to come.

For you, some of the recipes and ingredients will have immediate appeal, and others you may wrinkle your nose at—just play around until you get into your own GL groove, so to speak.

Don't forget that if you need more help and guidance you can take a look at www.dietfreedom.co.uk to check out the many services we provide to keep you bang up to date on GL and healthy eating.

In all the recipes, tsp = teaspoon, tbsp = tablespoon, and dsp = dessert spoon.

You will find GL estimates per serving for all recipes; these are estimates because precise GL scores for each recipe would need to be determined in a clinical study. So use these estimates as a guide—we don't expect you to start adding up your daily GL score.

This is "diet freedom" after all!

Chapter 9

FAST AND FRIENDLY RECIPES

Breakfast

Melon and Orange Smoothie

Preparation: 5 minutes, Serves 1

Estimated GL: 11

½ small melon, peeled, deseeded and chopped
1 large orange, peeled and chopped (pips removed)
1 lime, juice only
handful of fresh mint (optional)
2 tbsp natural, sugar-free yogurt

Add all ingredients together, blend and serve.

Cranberry and Apricot Muesli

Preparation: 10 minutes, Serves 4

Estimated GL per serving: 14

½ cup oats
1 tbsp dried apricots
1 tbsp dried cranberries (sugar-free)
your choice of milk to serve

Combine all dry ingredients in a bowl. Add desired amount of milk and serve.

Cheesy Herby Eggs on Toast

Preparation: 5 minutes, Cooking: 5 minutes, Serves 2

Estimated GL per serving: 4

4 large free-range eggs

4 tbsp milk

1 tsp olive-oil spread

2 tbsp cream cheese

2 tbsp mixed herbs (chives, parsley, oregano or whatever you
    have)

freshly ground black pepper

2 slices of toasted soy and flaxseed or rye bread

Beat the eggs and milk in a bowl and add black pepper.
Heat olive-oil spread in a frying pan and add egg
mixture. Stir constantly with wooden spoon until the
eggs are set but still soft. Remove pan from heat and stir
in cream cheese, herbs and pepper. Serve on the toasted
bread.

Watermelon Smoothie

Preparation: 5 minutes, Serves 1

Estimated GL: 6

¼ of a deseeded watermelon cut into chunks
handful of ice cubes
1 tbsp natural, sugar-free yogurt
2 tsp agave syrup
½ tsp ground ginger

Blend all ingredients together and serve.

Cinnamon and Chocolate Oatmeal

Preparation: 2 minutes, Cooking: 1–5 minutes depending on method used, Serves 1

Estimated GL: 12

2 tbsp oats
½ tsp cinnamon
2 tbsp water
1 tsp cocoa
1 tsp agave syrup
1 tsp boiling water

Place oatmeal and cinnamon in a microwave-safe bowl. Add water. Microwave on full power for 1 minute and stir. Add more water if necessary. Mix cocoa with agave syrup and boiling water to form a chocolate sauce. Drizzle over oatmeal. If preferred, you can cook the oatmeal on the stove in a small saucepan.

Nutty Blueberry Smoothie

Preparation: 10 minutes, Serves 2

Estimated GL per serving: 17

4 peaches or nectarines, sliced and pitted
½ cup blueberries, fresh or frozen
½ cup strawberries, fresh or frozen
1 large slightly unripe banana, cut into chunks
6 tbsp natural, sugar-free yogurt
6 Brazil nuts
2 tsp agave syrup

Place the peaches or nectarines into a juicer and extract the juice. Pour the juice into a blender with the remaining ingredients except the agave syrup and blend. Add agave syrup to sweeten if desired. Serve immediately in tall glasses.

Coconut and Apricot Energy Shake

Preparation: 5 minutes, Serves 1

Estimated GL: 9

½ cup coconut milk (no added sugar)
½ cup natural, sugar-free yogurt
handful dried apricots, chopped
handful ice
2 tsp agave syrup
¼–⅓ cup your choice of milk

Place all ingredients into a food processor or blender and blend together until combined and smooth. Pour into a tall serving glass and serve at once.

Lunch

Tuna and Bean Oatcakes

Preparation: 5 minutes, Serves 1

Estimated GL: 12

2 tbsp kidney beans
1 small can tuna, drained
½ red onion, diced
1 small tomato, diced
handful chopped fresh parsley (optional) or ½ tsp dried
1 tbsp pine nuts, toasted or untoasted
squeeze of fresh lemon juice
2 sugar-free oatcakes or Ryvita

Mix all together, squeeze over the lemon and serve with a couple of sugar-free oatcakes or Ryvita.

Wild Mushroom Omelette

Preparation: 5 minutes, Cooking: 20 minutes, Serves 2

Estimated GL per serving: 0

1 tbsp olive oil
2 cups wild mushrooms (or button)
4 large free-range eggs, beaten
freshly ground black pepper
1 cup any hard cheese, grated coarsely
parsley to taste

Heat half the oil in a pan, add the mushrooms and cook for 5 minutes until golden brown; set aside. Heat the rest of the oil in the same pan and add half of the beaten egg. Add black pepper and stir with a wooden spoon, bringing the cooked egg to the center and allowing the runny egg to go to the edge of the pan and cook. Add ½ of the mushrooms, cheese and parsley and fold omelette over, making sure egg is cooked through. Place on a warm serving plate and repeat process to make two omelettes.

Pumpkin and Coconut Soup

Preparation: 10 minutes, Cooking: 20 minutes, Serves 4

Estimated GL per serving: 6

1 red onion, chopped

1 tsp dried ginger

1 clove garlic, chopped or ½ tsp dried or purée

1 tsp olive oil

2.2 lb pumpkin, peeled and chopped

1½ cups organic vegetable stock

2 cups coconut milk (sugar-free)

freshly ground black pepper

Fry the onion, ginger and garlic in the olive oil until softened. Add the pumpkin and cover and steam on medium heat for about 10 minutes, stirring occasionally. Add the stock and coconut milk and cook until soft, adding more water if required. Add black pepper, blend until smooth and serve.

Tuna and Red Pepper Bowl

Preparation: 10 minutes, Serves 2

Estimated GL per serving: 6

1½ cups mixed beans
1 small can tuna, drained
1 red pepper, chopped
½ red onion, chopped
1 tbsp sundried tomatoes, chopped
1 tbsp extra virgin olive oil
1 tbsp red wine vinegar
freshly ground black pepper

Drain beans and tuna and mix with red pepper, onion and tomatoes. Combine olive oil, vinegar and black pepper for dressing. Combine altogether and serve in a bowl.

Broccoli and Almond Soup

Preparation: 5 minutes, Cooking: 15 minutes, Serves 4

Estimated GL per serving: 1

1 onion, chopped

2 leeks, chopped

1 garlic clove, crushed or ½ tsp dried/purée

Approx. 1lb. broccoli florets

1.5 liters organic vegetable stock

4 tbsp flaked almonds, toasted

4 tbsp crème fraîche

Fry onion, leeks and garlic in oil until softened. Add broccoli florets and 1.5 liters vegetable stock. Bring to boil and simmer until soft. Blend soup until smooth. Serve with toasted almonds and a spoonful of crème fraîche.

Perky Egg and Asparagus

Preparation: 10 minutes, Cooking: 8 minutes, Serves 2

Estimated GL per serving: 0

12 asparagus spears
water
½ tbsp white wine vinegar
4 large free-range eggs
4 tbsp olive oil–based spread
1 lemon, juice only
1 tbsp chopped fresh tarragon or 1 tsp dried/purée

Steam or boil asparagus for about 3 minutes or until just tender. Bring a pan of water to a boil and add the vinegar. Crack eggs in and simmer for a few minutes. Melt the spread in a pan and stir in the lemon juice and tarragon. Place asparagus spears on a plate, top with poached eggs, drizzle with the warm lemon and tarragon dressing and serve.

Bacon Frittata

Preparation: 5 minutes, Cooking: 10 minutes, Serves 1

Estimated GL per serving: 0

2 large free-range eggs
1 spring onion, chopped
1 tomato, chopped
freshly ground black pepper
drizzle of olive oil
2 slices lean bacon, chopped

Preheat oven to 425°F. Beat the eggs in a bowl and mix in the spring onion, tomato and seasoning. Heat the oil in a non-stick ovenproof frying pan and fry the bacon for a few minutes, until golden. Pour the egg mixture into a pan and evenly distribute mixture in pan. Cook until set and transfer to the oven for 4–5 minutes, until golden brown and cooked through. Remove from the oven and serve.

Dinner

Halloumi Cheese Kebabs

Preparation: 10 minutes, Cooking: 15 minutes, Serves 2

Estimated GL per serving: 2

1 tbsp agave syrup
1 tsp mustard
1 tbsp olive oil
½ lb. (usually one packet) halloumi cheese, cut into cubes
8 cherry tomatoes
8 button mushrooms
1 red onion, peeled, quartered

Preheat oven to 400°F. Mix together agave, mustard and olive oil. Thread the cheese, tomatoes, mushrooms and onion onto four metal skewers, alternating. Brush the agave/mustard mix over the skewered cheese and vegetables. Place on a baking tray, turning occasionally, and bake for up to 15 minutes or until golden brown.

Buckwheat Crepes with Smoked Salmon

Preparation: 10 minutes, Cooking: 10 minutes, Serves 2

Estimated GL per serving: 10

1 cup buckwheat flour

1 free-range egg

1 cup your choice of milk

½ cup ricotta cheese

1 garlic clove, crushed or ½ tsp dried/purée

2 tbsp chopped parsley

freshly ground black pepper

grated rind of half a lemon

2 tbsp olive oil

13.75 oz. can artichoke hearts, drained and chopped

juice of 1 lemon

½ lb. smoked salmon, cut into strips

Place the flour, egg and a splash of milk in a bowl and whisk until smooth. Gradually whisk in the remaining milk. Mix the ricotta with the garlic, parsley, pepper and lemon rind. Heat 1 tsp of the oil in a non-stick frying pan; when hot, pour off any excess and spoon 3 tbsp of the flour-and-milk batter into the pan. Cook on each side until browned. Transfer to a plate and keep warm. Make three more crepes in the same way, adding more oil if necessary. Divide the ricotta and artichoke between the crepes, drizzle with lemon juice, grind some black pepper over and serve with the salmon.

Salmon with Tomato and Lime Sauce

Preparation: 5 minutes, Cooking: 8 minutes, Serves 4

Estimated GL per serving: 1

½ tbsp olive oil

4 large boneless salmon fillets

2 tomatoes, finely chopped

½ red onion, finely chopped

juice and zest of 3 limes

2 tbsp chives, snipped

freshly ground black pepper

Heat the olive oil in a pan and cook the salmon for 4 minutes each side until cooked through. Mix the tomatoes, onion, lime juice, zest and chives together in a bowl and add black pepper. Place the salmon on plates, drizzle with the sauce and serve.

Quick Cajun Chicken

Preparation: 5 minutes, Cooking: 15 minutes, Serves 4

Estimated GL per serving: 0

1 tbsp paprika
½ tsp mild chili powder
4 skinless chicken breasts
1 tbsp olive oil

Preheat oven to 400°F. Mix together spices. Toss in chicken breasts and coat lightly. Drizzle oil over a baking sheet and add chicken breasts. Bake for 15 minutes or until cooked through.

Tuna Steak with Butter Beans

Preparation: 5 minutes, Cooking: 8 minutes, Serves 2

Estimated GL per serving: 4

2 cups (1 can) butterbeans, cooked
1 red onion, sliced
1 clove garlic crushed or ½ tsp powder/purée
1 tbsp extra virgin olive oil
2 tsp red wine vinegar
2 tuna steaks

Combine the butter beans, onion, garlic, olive oil and vinegar and set aside. Brush tuna with olive oil and fry for 4 minutes each side. Arrange butterbean salad on two plates and top with tuna steaks.

Steak, Mushroom and Red Pepper Stir-fry

Preparation: 5 minutes, Cooking: 15 minutes, Serves 4

Estimated GL per serving: 1

1 lb lean beef steak

1 tbsp olive oil

2 red peppers, deseeded and chopped

4 cups mushrooms, sliced

1 clove garlic, crushed or ½ tsp dried/purée

1 cup snow peas

⅔ cup crème fraîche

1 tsp whole grain mustard

Cut steak into strips and fry in the preheated oil in a large frying pan or wok for about 5 minutes until the meat starts to brown. Add red pepper, mushrooms and garlic. Cook for a few minutes until softened. Add the snow peas, crème fraîche and mustard, stir and cook for a few more minutes.

Pork with Mustard Sauce and Pasta

Preparation: 10 minutes, Cooking: 10 minutes, Serves 2

Estimated GL per serving: 9

4 cups buckwheat, whole grain or chickpea pasta
1 tbsp olive oil
1 red onion, chopped
1 red pepper, deseeded and sliced
2 large lean pork medallions, trimmed and sliced
1 cup crème fraîche or single cream
2 tsp whole grain mustard
freshly ground black pepper
water as needed

Boil pasta with a tsp of the olive oil in boiling water until just cooked but still firm to the bite (*al dente*). Drain pasta and set aside. Heat olive oil in a large frying pan. Add onion and red pepper until they start to soften. Add pork, stirring until brown and cooked through. Stir in crème fraîche, mustard and black pepper. Add some water to thin down the sauce. Stir in pasta and serve.

Chapter 10

VEGGIE-FRIENDLY RECIPES

Breakfast

"Feelin' Fruity" Yog-bowl

Preparation: 5 minutes, Serves 2

Estimated GL per serving: 8

⅔ cup chopped mixed nuts
1 cup natural, sugar-free yogurt
1 apple, finely diced
2 tbsp dried cranberries (sugar-free), chopped

Mix all ingredients together in a bowl and serve.

Banana and Strawberry Smoothie

Preparation: 5 minutes, Serves 1

Estimated GL: 8

1 slightly unripe frozen banana, cut into chunks
½ cup natural, sugar-free yogurt
2½ cups fresh strawberries
grated nutmeg (optional)

Combine all ingredients except nutmeg in a blender and purée until smooth and creamy. Pour into a glass and dust with nutmeg.

Apple and Hazelnut Muesli

Preparation: 10 minutes, Serves 4

Estimated GL per serving: 20

½ cup rolled oats
½ cup dried apricots, roughly chopped
½ cup toasted hazelnuts, chopped roughly
1 cup fresh apple juice
2 apples, peeled and grated
1 cup natural, sugar-free yogurt
1 tbsp agave syrup

In a large bowl mix together the oats, apricots and hazelnuts. Pour over the apple juice and leave for 10 minutes to allow the oats and dried fruit to soak up the juice. Divide the muesli between 4 bowls and top with grated apple. Spoon on a dollop of yogurt and drizzle over agave syrup. Serve immediately.

Apricot and Almond Smoothie

Preparation: 5 minutes, Serves 2

Estimated GL per serving: 12

6 fresh apricots (or tinned in natural juice—not syrup)
1 cup fresh orange juice with pulp
1 cup natural, sugar-free yogurt
1 tsp ground flax seeds (optional)
2 tbsp flaked almonds
grated nutmeg (optional)

Throw everything together, blend and serve.

Pear and Pumpkin Seed Yog-bowl

Preparation: 5 minutes, Serves 1

Estimated GL: 6

1 large firm pear, chopped

1 tbsp Greek yogurt or natural thick yogurt

1 tbsp pumpkin seeds (toasted if preferred)

Combine the yogurt and pear. Sprinkle over the pumpkin seeds and serve.

Tofu and Sunflower Smoothie

Preparation: 5 minutes, Serves 1

Estimated GL: 13

½ cup soft tofu

1 apple, chopped

1 cup your choice of milk

1 tbsp sunflower seeds

1 tsp unsweetened cocoa powder

2 tsp agave syrup

Throw everything together, blend and serve.

Hot Apple Oatmeal

Preparation: 1 minute, Cooking: 1 minute, Serves 1

Estimated GL: 16

2 tbsp oats
1 large apple, finely chopped or grated
½ cup water
1 tbsp natural, sugar-free yogurt

Place oatmeal in a microwave-safe bowl. Add water and apple and stir. Microwave on full power for 1 minute and stir. Add more water if necessary. Top with yogurt and serve. If preferred, you can cook the oatmeal on the stove in a small saucepan.

Lunch

Fennel Soup

Preparation: 10 minutes, Cooking: 35 minutes, Serves 4—6

Estimated GL: 0

1 medium onion, chopped
2 tbsp olive oil
4 bulbs fennel, chopped
bouquet garni—3 parsley stalks, 1 sprig thyme, 1 bay leaf, tied
    together
3½ cups organic vegetable stock
freshly ground black pepper

To garnish:
fennel leaves
lemon zest

In a large pan, fry the onion in olive oil for approximately
5 minutes until translucent. Stir in the fennel and add the
bouquet garni, stock and pepper. Bring to the boil, cover
and simmer for 30 minutes until the vegetables are very
tender. Remove the bouquet garni and allow the soup to
cool slightly. Blend the soup until it is smooth, either with
a hand blender or in a blender. Reheat. Garnish with the
fennel leaves and lemon zest and serve immediately.

Endive with Watercress and Orange Salad

Preparation: 10 minutes, Serves 4

Estimated GL per serving: 4

3 heads endive
3 large oranges
2 bunches watercress
3 tbsp extra virgin olive oil or peanut oil
freshly ground black pepper

Trim the endive, separate into leaves, wash and dry. Put into a salad bowl. Coarsely grate (or use a zester) the zest of one orange, place in a small bowl. Squeeze the juice and add to the zest. Peel the remaining 2 oranges and cut into segments (make sure you have no pith on the segments). Add the orange to the chicory. Trim, wash and add the watercress to the salad. Add the oil and black pepper to the orange zest and juice and whisk together. Pour over the salad, toss and serve immediately.

Spinach, Avocado, Pea and Mint Salad

Preparation: 10 minutes, Serves 2

Estimated GL per serving: 3

1 large bag fresh spinach leaves, rinsed and dried
1 large avocado, skinned, pitted and cut into chunks
1½ cups peas—fresh or frozen and defrosted
1 generous handful of fresh mint
2 tbsp avocado oil or extra virgin olive oil
1 tbsp white wine vinegar
freshly ground black pepper
small handful of pumpkin seeds

Put the spinach, avocado, peas and fresh mint into a salad bowl. Whisk the oil, vinegar and black pepper together. Pour over the salad leaves and toss well. In a small frying pan, heat the pumpkin seeds over a high heat until they "pop" and turn golden. Sprinkle over the salad, serve immediately. (If you don't have fresh mint, add a teaspoon of dried mint to the dressing.)

Grilled Asparagus with Fresh Mint and Feta Cheese

Preparation: 5 minutes, Cooking: 4–5 minutes, Serves 2

Estimated GL per serving: 0

12 fresh asparagus spears
2 tbsp lemon juice
2 tbsp olive oil
freshly ground black pepper
½ cup feta cheese
2 tsp fresh mint leaves, roughly chopped

Preheat grill to a high heat. Trim the woody ends off the asparagus and place on a heat-proof plate. Mix 1 tbsp of lemon juice and 1 tbsp of olive oil and the black pepper together and pour over the asparagus. Place the plate under the grill, turning occasionally, for about 4–5 minutes. Pour any juice left on the plate into a jar; add the rest of the olive oil and lemon juice and more black pepper to taste, put the lid on the jar and shake into a dressing. Cut the feta into chunks. Arrange the cooked asparagus and feta between the two plates, sprinkle with mint, and pour over the dressing. Serve immediately. (If you don't have fresh mint add a teaspoon of dried mint to the dressing.)

Spinach and Cheese Soufflé

Preparation: 5 minutes, Cooking: 40 minutes, Serves 4

Estimated GL per serving: 3

2 tbsp olive oil–based spread

1 tbsp spelt flour

¾ cup your choice of milk

3 large free-range eggs, separated

1 cup frozen spinach, thawed and squeezed dry

1 cup sharp Cheddar cheese, coarsely grated

¼ tsp grated nutmeg

freshly ground black pepper

2 tbsp Parmesan cheese, grated

Preheat oven to 375°F. Grease 4 large ramekin dishes (or one 6-inch/15-cm soufflé dish) and tie a paper "collar" round each to support the soufflé as it rises. Melt the olive oil–based spread in a small pan, stir in the flour and cook for a minute. Remove from heat and stir in the milk, return to the heat and slowly bring to the boil, stirring all the time. Cook for 3 minutes, then take off the heat and add the egg yolks, spinach, Cheddar, nutmeg, pepper and half the Parmesan and mix thoroughly. Whisk the egg whites until fairly stiff. Using a metal spoon, fold one spoonful of the egg white mix into the spinach mix, then carefully fold in the rest. Transfer to the prepared dishes, sprinkle with the remaining Parmesan cheese. Bake for 15–20 minutes (25–30 minutes if in one large dish) until risen and golden. Serve immediately with a green salad.

No-fuss Lentil Soup

Preparation: 10 minutes, Cooking: 45 minutes, Serves 4

Estimated GL per serving: 2

2 tbsp olive oil

1 medium onion, chopped

2 medium carrots, chopped

3 sticks celery, chopped

1 clove garlic, chopped or grated

4 cardamom pods, split but with seeds left in

1 cup dried lentils

2½ cups organic vegetable stock

freshly ground black pepper

fresh parsley to garnish

Heat the oil in large pan, add the vegetables (these or any you like best) and garlic and fry until softened. Add the remaining ingredients. Bring to a boil, cover and simmer for 45 minutes, stirring occasionally. Check the seasoning and serve sprinkled with parsley.

Spicy Aduki Bean Soup

Preparation: 15 minutes, Cooking: 1 hour 15 minutes, Serves 4

Estimated GL per serving: 3

1 cup aduki beans, soaked for 3 hours in cold water
2 tbsp olive oil
1 medium onion, chopped
2 tbsp hot pepper sauce
3 sticks of celery, chopped
2 medium carrots, chopped
2 cloves garlic, chopped or grated
½ 14.5-oz can of tomatoes
1 tbsp tomato purée
1 bay leaf
1 tsp fresh thyme, chopped
3½ cups organic vegetable stock
freshly ground black pepper
handful of fresh parsley, chopped (optional)

Once the beans have been soaking in cold water for 3 hours, drain and rinse. Heat the oil in a large pan, add the onion, harissa paste, celery, carrots and garlic and cook until the vegetables start to soften. Add all the remaining ingredients except the parsley. Bring to a boil and cook on a high heat for 10 minutes, then simmer gently for an hour. Serve with freshly chopped parsley if desired.

Dinner

Spicy Tofu

Preparation: 5 minutes, Cooking: 10 minutes, Serves 2

Estimated GL per serving: 3

1 cup firm organic tofu
1 tsp olive oil
2 tsp sesame seed oil
2 tbsp soy sauce
1 tsp Chinese 5 spice
2 tsp agave syrup
a few sesame seeds for sprinkling over finished dish
low-GL vegetables to stir-fry or steam

Slice tofu into 1-inch-thick slices and dry with kitchen paper. Heat olive oil in a pan, add tofu and cook on both sides for about 10 minutes until it turns golden brown. Combine sesame oil, soy sauce and spices in a bowl. Add the warm tofu, then add the sesame seeds and stir well. Drizzle over the agave syrup and sprinkle a few sesame seeds on top. Serve with steamed or stir-fried vegetables.

Eastern Vegetables

Preparation: 20 minutes, Cooking: 20 minutes, Serves 6

Estimated GL per serving: 9

2 generous cups couscous

2 tbsp peanut oil

2 tsp curry powder

1 tsp cumin seeds

1 large onion, sliced

2 small sweet potatoes, peeled and cubed

4 carrots, sliced

2 cups cauliflower florets

approx. 6 dried apricots, cut into chunks

½ cup water

1 generous handful fresh cilantro, roughly chopped

zest of 1 lemon, grated

Cook the couscous as per the packet instructions. Put the oil into a large saucepan (with lid), add the curry powder, cumin seeds and onion, cook until the onion is soft. Add the vegetables, apricots and the water, bring to a boil, cover and simmer until tender. Drain any excess water from the couscous, stir in the cilantro and lemon zest. Serve with the vegetables. If you like, choose your favorite fresh herb to stir into the couscous.

Hot and Spicy Vegetable Stir-fry with Coconut Milk

Preparation: 10 minutes, Cooking: 10 minutes, Serves 6

Estimated GL per serving: 2

2 pieces lemongrass

1 tsp cumin seeds

4 fresh red chilies, deseeded and finely chopped

2-inch piece fresh ginger, peeled and finely diced, or 1 tsp
     dried/purée

4 cups mixed vegetables, such as broccoli, cauliflower florets,
     eggplant, asparagus, carrot, sugar snaps, sweet potato,
     zucchini—all cut into slices/chunks roughly the same size

2 tbsp peanut oil

1 cup coconut milk (no added sugar)

Trim off the root end of the lemongrass and finely chop the more tender part of the stalk. Crush the cumin seeds and add the finely chopped chilies and ginger. Mix together to form a paste, preferably with a pestle and mortar (though you can also use a small blender to chop and blend the spicy chili mixture. You may also want to add lime leaves or cardamom seeds to the spice blend). Once your vegetables and chili paste are ready, heat the oil in a large frying pan or wok over a medium heat. Add the chili mixture and, stirring continuously, fry for 3–4 minutes. Add the coconut milk and bring to the boil, then add all the vegetables and cook for 5–6 minutes until they are starting to become tender. Serve immediately on warm plates.

Spicy Vegetable Dal

Preparation: 20 minutes, Cooking: 1hr 10 minutes, Serves 4

Estimated GL per serving: 3

1 cup yellow split peas (dal)

3½ cups water

2 large carrots, sliced

½ small cauliflower, cut into florets/chunks

1 medium zucchini, thickly sliced

1 tbsp peanut oil

1 large onion, finely chopped

2 garlic cloves, chopped or grated

1 tsp ground coriander

5 whole cardamom pods

1 tsp freshly grated ginger, or ½ tsp dried

Rinse split peas and put into a large saucepan, cover with cold water and bring to the boil. Simmer for about 1 hour or until the peas start to soften—topping up the water as necessary to keep them covered. Add the carrots, cauliflower and zucchini and simmer until tender—approximately 10 minutes. Heat the oil in the frying pan; cook the onion until softening, stir in the garlic and spices, and cook for a further 3–4 minutes. Drain the split pea and veggie mix, then stir in the onion and spices.

Bulgur and Butternut Squash

Preparation: 10 minutes, Cooking: 20 minutes, Serves 2

Estimated GL per serving: 12

2¼ lb butternut squash, peeled and diced

1¼ cups of bulgur wheat, cooked as per instructions on
    packet

1¼ cups feta cheese, cubed

handful of fresh sage, chopped or ½ tsp dried freshly ground
    black pepper

1 tbsp agave syrup

juice of 1 lemon

Roast butternut squash in oven, covered, at 350°F until just starting to soften. Combine the cooked bulgur wheat, feta and roasted squash. Add the chopped sage and black pepper and toss together. Combine agave syrup with lemon juice, drizzle over and serve.

Squash also goes well with cinnamon, chili, coriander and nutmeg.

Beanie Casserole

Preparation: 15 minutes, Cooking: 25 minutes, Serves 4

Estimated GL per serving: 20

1 onion, chopped

1 clove garlic, chopped or ½ tsp dried/purée

2½–3 cups button mushrooms, sliced

1 leek, chopped

1 tbsp olive oil

2 generous cups mixed beans

16 oz can red kidney beans

2 16 oz cans/4 generous cups chopped tomatoes

2 tbsp Parmesan cheese, grated

2 small parsnips, peeled and grated

Preheat oven to 400°F. Fry onion, garlic, mushrooms and leek in a pan in the olive oil until softened. Rinse and drain assorted beans and kidney beans and add to pan. Add tomatoes and heat through. Combine the Parmesan and the grated parsnip. Place the bean mixture in an ovenproof casserole dish. Cover with the Parmesan and parsnip mixture and sprinkle over some olive oil. Bake for 25 minutes or until golden brown and crispy.

Cheese and Mushroom Tortilla

Preparation: 10 minutes, Cooking: 35 minutes, Serves 4

Estimated GL per serving: 9

2 tbsp olive oil

2 medium sweet potatoes, peeled and diced

4–5 cups button mushrooms, sliced

1 leek, sliced

6 large free-range eggs

handful fresh chives, chopped or 1 tsp dried

3 cups mature Cheddar cheese (or any hard cheese), coarsely grated

Heat the oil in a medium-size pan over a medium heat. Add potatoes and cook for 5 minutes until turning golden. Add mushrooms and leek and cook until softened. Meanwhile, beat the eggs together in a bowl with 2 tbsp cold water. Add chives and cheese and pour into the pan. Cover pan and cook for 15 minutes on a low heat, tilting pan so that uncooked mixture runs to the outside and cooks. The tortilla should be set throughout and golden underneath. Divide into 4 slices and serve warm.

Chapter 11

FOODIE-FRIENDLY RECIPES

Breakfast

Orange Spice Oatmeal

Preparation: 5 minutes, Cooking: 5 minutes (microwave), 10 minutes (stove), Serves 1

Estimated GL per serving: 12

2 level tbsp oats

½ cup water

1 tsp cinnamon

1 tsp ground ginger (or fresh grated ginger)

zest of half an orange

1 tbsp freshly squeezed orange juice (or orange juice not from
   concentrate)

1 tsp agave syrup

1 tbsp crème fraîche

If using microwave:

Put the oats, water, cinnamon, ginger, orange zest and juice in a microwaveable bowl, cook for approximately 3 minutes and stir. Return to cook for a bit longer if necessary. Stir in the agave syrup, and dollop on the crème fraîche.

If using stove:

Cook the oats, water and cinnamon in a small saucepan over a high heat, stirring continuously until it reaches the desired consistency. Stir in the agave syrup, and dollop on the crème fraîche.

You can use fructose to sweeten if you don't have agave.

Mushroom "Toast" with Scrambled Eggs and Smoky Bacon

Preparation: 5 minutes, Cooking: 15 minutes, Serves 2

Estimated GL per serving: 0

4 slices lean bacon
2 large flat mushrooms, stalks removed
1 tbsp olive oil–based spread
4 free-range eggs
freshly ground black pepper

Heat the grill to medium. Put the bacon and mushrooms (top facing up) under the grill. Carefully take the mushrooms out when starting to brown on top, turn over and spread the underside of mushrooms with half the spread, put back under the grill topside-down until mushrooms start to brown and bacon is cooked. Meanwhile, whisk together the eggs with the black pepper in a bowl. Place a small saucepan on medium heat, add the remaining spread, and when melted add the egg mixture. Stir eggs continuously with a wooden spoon until just scrambled. Take off the heat and fill the underside of the mushrooms with the scrambled egg. Chop the cooked bacon, sprinkle over the eggy mushrooms and serve.

Sweet and Savory "No Cook" Breakfast

Preparation: 7 minutes, Serves 1

Estimated GL per serving: 4

1 generous slice watermelon, cut into chunks
1 matchbox-size piece Jarlsberg cheese (or any cheese you
     have), cubed
1 thick slice of ham, cut into strips (from deli counter—not
     "plastic" ham!)
5 strawberries, washed, hulled and halved
handful of blueberries, washed
1 tsp balsamic vinegar

Arrange a layer of watermelon on a plate. Sprinkle the ham and the cheese cubes over the top. Top with the strawberries and blueberries. Drizzle balsamic vinegar over the top and serve.

Chocolate Smoothie

Preparation: 7 minutes, Serves 1

Estimated GL per serving: 10

water
your choice of milk
1 heaped tsp cocoa (unsweetened)
1 medium firm banana, cut into chunks
1 tsp fresh grated ginger (or ½ tsp ground ginger)
1 tsp flaxseed
1 tsp agave syrup (optional)

Using the glass you'll drink your smoothie from, measure the water and milk out, adding half and half so the glass is ¾ full, and add to the blender. Add all other ingredients, blend until smooth and serve.

Apricot "Jam" on Toast

Preparation: 5 minutes, Cooking: 10 minutes, Serves 4 servings of "jam" which will keep in the fridge for a few days

Estimated GL per serving: 5

½ cup dried apricots
2 tbsp water
1 tsp agave syrup or fructose
1 slice of low-GL toast (such as soy and flaxseed)

Chop the dried apricots into very small pieces. Put the apricots, water and syrup/fructose into a small saucepan and bring to the boil. Boil rapidly for a few minutes, but don't let it boil dry! Take off the heat and allow to cool. Spread on the toast. Put the remainder of the cooled jam in a covered pot in the fridge. This jam is also good stirred into yogurt, or to add a bit of sweetness to oatmeal or muesli.

Cheesy Puffs

**Preparation: 10 minutes, Cooking: 10 minutes,
Serves 4 (2 puffs each)**

Estimated GL per serving: 0

4 free-range egg whites
½ cup ground almonds
½ tsp cream of tartar
2 tbsp fresh Parmesan cheese, finely grated
2 tbsp strong Cheddar, coarsely grated, or any other hard
    cheese
1 tsp paprika

Preheat oven to 350°F. Grease a deep muffin tin, or use
muffin cases. Whisk the egg whites until stiff and glossy.
Mix the ground almonds, cream of tartar, cheeses and
paprika together in a bowl. Gradually fold the cheese
mixture into the egg whites, gently. Divide the mixture
between the 8 tins/cases. Bake for 10 minutes or until
golden. Remove from oven and place on a wire rack to
cool slightly.

These are lovely warm, but also very good cold for a
lunchbox-filler.

Zesty Yog-bowl

Preparation: 5 minutes, Serves 1

Estimated GL per serving: 5

3 tbsp natural, sugar-free yogurt
zest of 1 lemon
2 tbsp your favorite toasted seeds
1 tsp agave syrup

Place all ingredients into a bowl, combine and serve.

Lunch

Zucchini and Mackerel Stir-fry

Preparation: 10 minutes, Cooking: 10 minutes, Serves 1

Estimated GL per serving: 5

1 tbsp olive oil
1 small zucchini, washed and sliced into rounds
freshly ground black pepper
4 cherry tomatoes, halved
¼ cup chickpeas, drained and rinsed
1 garlic clove, chopped or grated or ½ tsp dried or purée
1 small can (¾ cup) mackerel in tomato sauce
dash of Tabasco sauce

Heat the oil in a frying pan on high heat. Add the zucchini, grind over the black pepper and cook for a minute or so on each side until starting to soften. Add the tomatoes, chickpeas and garlic and cook for another minute or so until all tender. Turn down the heat, stir in the mackerel and Tabasco and heat through. Take off the heat and serve immediately.

You can stir in some fresh herbs such as basil and/or grate over a little Parmesan cheese.

Hot Dressed Salad

Preparation: 10 minutes, Cooking: 10 minutes, Serves 2

Estimated GL per serving: 0

2 small heads Romaine lettuce
1 lime
1 tsp olive oil
1 garlic clove, chopped or grated, or ½ tsp dried or purée
6 slices lean bacon
freshly ground black pepper

Wash and dry the lettuce, and arrange in a serving dish. Coarsely grate the lime (or use a zester), squeeze the juice from the lime and reserve. Heat the oil in a pan and add the garlic and bacon, frying until bacon is crispy. Discard any excess rind and finely chop the bacon. In a bowl, add the lime juice to the bacon and stir to combine. Pour the bacon mixture over the leaves and toss to coat. Sprinkle with lime zest and pepper; serve immediately.

You could add some grilled sliced chicken breast to the salad.

Chicken, Avocado and Arugula Wrap

Preparation: 10 minutes, Serves 2

Estimated GL per serving: 10

1 ready-grilled or roasted skinless chicken breast

1 avocado, peeled, pitted and cut into chunks

1 tbsp mayonnaise

1 tbsp fresh lemon juice

freshly ground black pepper

handful of arugula, washed and dried

2 stoneground wholemeal tortilla wraps

Cut the chicken into slices on the diagonal and put to one side. Put the avocado, mayonnaise, lemon juice and pepper into a bowl and roughly mash together. Divide the avocado mixture between the two wraps, add some arugula and the chicken. Wrap and serve.

Herby Mussels

Preparation: 5 minutes, Cooking: 15 minutes, Serves 2

Estimated GL per serving: 2

4.4 lb fresh mussels
2 cups dry white wine or dry sherry
2 cloves garlic, chopped or grated
handful fresh parsley, chopped
small handful fresh dill, chopped
small handful fresh chives, chopped
chopped herbs to garnish (reserve from above)
4 tbsp olive oil–based spread
2 tbsp Parmesan cheese, grated

Place the mussels and all ingredients (except the Parmesan) into a large saucepan with a lid. Pour over the wine, bring to boil, cover and cook until the shells have opened—approximately 5–10 minutes. Discard any mussels that haven't opened. Transfer to a serving dish, sprinkle with Parmesan, garnish with herbs and serve.

Robust "Root" Soup

Preparation: 10 minutes, Cooking: 10 minutes, Serves 4

Estimated GL per serving: 6

1 onion, chopped

2 garlic cloves, chopped or grated or 1 tsp dried or purée

2 tsp olive oil

1 carrot, peeled and chopped

1 sweet potato, peeled and chopped

1 turnip, peeled and chopped

1 parsnip, peeled and chopped

1 tsp ground ginger

half tsp dried chili flakes

5 cups organic vegetable stock

Fry onion and garlic in olive oil in a large pan for a few minutes until softened. Add all root vegetables and cook for about 10 minutes until softened. Add ginger and chili flakes and cover with vegetable stock. Cook for 10 minutes, blend and serve.

Salmon and Cherry Tomato Frittata

Preparation: 5 minutes, Cooking: 8 minutes, Serves 2

Estimated GL per serving: 2

2 tbsp olive oil

8 spring onions, sliced

1 garlic clove, chopped or grated or half tsp dried or purée

10 cherry tomatoes, halved

4 large free-range eggs

small bunch fresh mint, chopped (optional)

freshly ground black pepper

1 cup red salmon, drained, skin and bones removed

1 cup frozen peas, defrosted and drained

Heat the oil in a non-stick frying pan and fry the spring onions and garlic for a few minutes. Add the tomatoes. Beat the eggs with the mint, season with pepper and swirl the egg mixture into the pan. Scatter over the flaked salmon and the peas and cook over a medium heat for 3–4 minutes until almost set. Carefully cook under a preheated grill for a further 2–3 minutes until lightly browned on top and cooked through. Serve warm, cut into wedges.

Rye Bread and Salmon Slices

Preparation: 15 minutes, Serves 2

Estimated GL per serving: 3

2 large free-range eggs

2 tsp creamed horseradish

2 slices 100 percent rye bread

1 little butter lettuce, washed

2 generous slices smoked salmon

1 tbsp mayonnaise

1 tsp fresh dill, chopped, or half a tsp of dried

few sprigs fresh dill to decorate (optional)

freshly ground black pepper

fresh lemon wedges to serve

Boil the eggs until hard-boiled, drain and place in cold water. Spread the horseradish on the rye bread and put each slice on a plate. Arrange some of the lettuce leaves on the bread. Lay the slices of salmon over the top. Peel and quarter the cooled hard-boiled eggs, and arrange on top of the salmon. Mix the fresh dill with the mayonnaise and spread over the top. Grind over black pepper to taste. Serve with lemon wedges.

Dinner

Garlic, Lemon and Cumin Pork Chops

Preparation: 10 minutes, Marinade: 2 hours,
Cooking: 15–20 minutes, Serves 4

Estimated GL per serving: 0

1 tsp cumin, ground
1 tsp cilantro seeds, ground
½ tsp chili powder
1 onion, roughly chopped
4 tbsp olive oil
juice and rind of half a lemon
4 large pork chops, fat removed
lemon wedges to serve

Place all the ingredients (except the pork and lemon wedges) into a blender and blend into a paste. Transfer into a sturdy freezer bag, add the pork chops and "squelch" until you are sure all the meat is well covered. Seal the bag, place in a bowl and refrigerate for at least 2 hours. When you're ready to cook, heat the grill to a high heat and grill the chops for 6–10 minutes each side, depending on thickness, until cooked through.

Serve with lemon wedges and low-GL veggies or a crunchy salad.

Great for the BBQ.

Spicy Yogurt Chicken

Preparation: 10 minutes, Cooking: 15–20 minutes, Serves 4

Estimated GL per serving: 1

1¼ cups natural, sugar-free yogurt
1 large onion, diced
2 garlic cloves, chopped or grated, or 1 tsp dried or purée
1 tsp cilantro seeds, crushed
handful fresh mint, chopped, or 1 tsp dried
1 tbsp cumin seeds, crushed
2 tbsp smoked paprika
zest of one lemon
4 large skinless chicken breasts
lemon wedges to serve

Combine all ingredients, except chicken and lemon wedges, in a bowl and mix well. Place mixture in a sturdy freezer bag. Add the chicken breasts and "squelch" until all the chicken breasts have a good covering. Seal the bag, place in a bowl and refrigerate for at least 2 hours, up to 24 hours. When you're ready to cook, heat the grill to a high heat. Grill the chicken for 6–10 minutes each side or until cooked through.

Serve with lemon wedges and low-GL veggies or a crispy salad.

Great for kebabs or the BBQ.

Beef Kebabs

Preparation: 30 minutes, Cooking: 20 minutes, Serves 4

Estimated GL per serving: 1

2 tbsp olive oil

2 tbsp white wine vinegar

4 dashes Tabasco sauce (or other pepper sauce)

1 clove garlic, chopped or grated

1½lb lean steak, cut into cubes

8 firm cherry tomatoes

1 red onion, cut into quarters

3 zucchini cut into chunky rounds

8 button mushrooms

Mix the olive oil, vinegar, Tabasco and garlic together in a bowl. Add the meat, toss to cover and allow to stand for 15 minutes. Thread 8 metal skewers, alternating the meat and veggies. Grill for 20 minutes, turning at least once, until meat is cooked through and vegetables are golden.

Great with salad and hummus.

Sweet Potato and Haddock Fishcakes

Preparation: 30 minutes, Cooking: 7 minutes, Serves 4

Estimated GL per serving: 12

4 boneless haddock fillets (or any white fish)
water
4 small sweet potatoes
2 tsp olive oil–based spread
handful fresh parsley, chopped
freshly ground black pepper
2 tsp grainy mustard
2 tbsp peanut oil

Poach the haddock in a large frying pan with enough water to cover the fish until cooked through. Remove from the water, allow to cool and flake into a large bowl. Boil sweet potatoes until just tender, drain and mash with the spread. Add the flaked haddock to the potato mash. Add parsley, pepper and mustard and combine well. Mold 8 fishcakes from this mixture. Heat the oil in a pan and fry fishcakes over a medium heat on both sides until crisp and golden. Drain well on kitchen paper.

Delicious with salad, tomato salsa and mayonnaise.

Chili Bean Cassoulet

Preparation: 10 minutes, Cooking: 10 minutes, Serves 6

Estimated GL per serving: 12

2 cups lean bacon, chopped
1 tbsp olive oil
2 generous cups chickpeas, drained and rinsed
1 cup butter beans, drained and rinsed
1 cup sweet corn, drained and rinsed
4 cups green beans (fresh or frozen), chopped
2 cups kidney beans, drained and rinsed
1 tsp chili powder
1 tsp paprika (smoked paprika is even better)
3 dashes Worcestershire sauce
2 dashes Tabasco sauce
¼ cup tomato purée
1⅓ cups organic vegetable or chicken stock

Fry the bacon in the olive oil in a large saucepan until crispy. Add the rest of the ingredients to the pan, bring to the boil and simmer for about 5 minutes and serve hot.

You can use any combination of beans.

You can use a different meat, or even fish.

Allow to go cold and use as a snack or lunchbox-filler.

Fish Curry with Rice and Beans

Preparation: 15 minutes, Cooking: 40 minutes, Serves 4

Estimated GL per serving: 12

For the rice and beans:

1⅓ cups brown rice

2 tbsp olive oil

1 onion, chopped

2 garlic cloves, chopped or 1 tsp dried or purée

2 generous cups chickpeas, drained and rinsed

zest of 1 lemon

For the curry:

approx. 1 lb boneless white fish steaks or fillets

4 tbsp peanut oil

1-inch piece fresh ginger, finely diced, or 1 tsp dried

2 garlic cloves, finely chopped, or 1 tsp dried or purée

4 shallots, peeled and chopped

1 tbsp garam masala (or 2 tsp cilantro seeds, 1½ tsp cumin
    seeds, 1 tsp fennel seeds, 3 cloves—ground together and
    mixed with 1 tsp ground cinnamon)

½ tsp hot chili flakes

freshly ground black pepper

1 tsp turmeric

1 tsp cayenne pepper

2 generous cups chopped tomatoes

⅔ cup organic vegetable stock or water

juice of half a lemon

handful cilantro, roughly chopped or 1 tsp dried

¾ cup natural, sugar-free yogurt

Cook the rice as per the packet instructions, drain and set aside. In a large pan, heat the olive oil over a medium heat and fry the onions for 5 minutes. Add the garlic, chickpeas and rice and stir-fry for a couple minutes. Stir in the lemon zest, set aside and keep warm to serve with the curry.

Cut the fish into 2-inch pieces. In a large frying pan, heat the oil over a high heat and fry the fish until no longer opaque. Place fish on a paper towel on a plate to remove excess oil. Turn the pan down to a medium heat, and add the ginger, garlic and shallots. Fry for 5 minutes, add the garam masala, chili flakes, black pepper, turmeric and cayenne and cook for another minute. Add the tomatoes and stock or water, stir and then add the lemon juice. Place the fish carefully back into the pan and cover with the sauce. Sprinkle with a few more chili flakes and simmer for about 10 minutes. Sprinkle the cilantro over the rice and beans and stir through. Arrange the rice and beans on serving plates. Spoon the curry over the rice and beans.

Add a spoonful of natural, sugar-free yogurt over the curry.

Kashmiri Chicken

Preparation: 10 minutes, Cooking: 35 minutes, Serves 6

Estimated GL per serving: 1

4 tbsp olive oil–based spread

2 tbsp olive oil

3 large onions, finely sliced

10 peppercorns

10 cardamom pods, split

2-inch cinnamon stick

2-inch piece of fresh ginger, chopped fine or 1 tsp dried

3 garlic cloves, finely chopped, or 1 ½ tsp dried or purée

1 tsp chili powder

1 tsp paprika

3.3 lb skinless chicken pieces

1 cup natural, sugar-free yogurt

Melt the spread and olive oil in a large frying pan with lid. Add the onions, peppercorns, cardamom and cinnamon and fry until the onions are golden. Add the ginger, garlic, chili powder and paprika and fry for a further 2 minutes, stirring. Add the chicken pieces and fry until starting to brown. Gradually add the yogurt, stirring constantly. Cover and cook gently until the chicken is cooked through—approximately 30 minutes.

Serve with couscous (with chopped fresh herbs and lemon zest stirred through it).

Serve with one of the marvellous mash recipes—see page 197.

Spicy Indian dishes are surprisingly lovely served with a crunchy iceberg lettuce salad.

Chapter 12

MORE LOW-GL RECIPES – FOOD THAT LOVES YOU BACK!

Now that you're getting in to the low-GL groove, here are some more delicious recipes.

We have given symbols to the recipes (see box below) so you can see at a glance how quick they are and if they are suitable for vegetarians.

Fast and Friendly—20 minutes or less to make

Veggie-friendly—suitable for vegetarians

Foodie-friendly—takes just a little bit more time and effort

More Breakfast Ideas

Smoked Salmon and Eggs with Rye Toast

Preparation: 10 minutes, Cooking: 7 minutes, Serves 2

Estimated GL per serving: 3

2 large free-range eggs at room temperature

2 slices rye bread

1 tsp olive oil–based spread

2 large slices smoked salmon

1 tsp capers, finely chopped

freshly ground black pepper

1 lemon, cut into wedges

Put the eggs into a small pan of water on the stove, bring to the boil and cook for approximately 7 minutes, until hard-boiled. Run under cold water and remove the shell. Toast the rye bread and spread thinly with olive oil–based spread. Drape the smoked salmon over toast and sprinkle with chopped capers. Cut eggs into slices and layer onto the toast. Grind over plenty of black pepper. Serve with lemon wedges on the side.

Sweet 'n' Nutty Toast

Preparation: 5 minutes, Serves 1

Estimated GL per serving: 10

1 slice low-GL bread

1 unpeeled apple, coarsely grated

1 pinch cinnamon

1 tsp agave syrup

1 tsp crunchy peanut butter (sugar-free)

Toast the bread. Mix all the ingredients together in a bowl, and spread onto the toast.

Crunchy Nectarine Granola

Preparation: 10 minutes, Serves 1

Estimated GL per serving: 8

1 nectarine, pitted and chopped
½ cup natural, sugar-free yogurt
2 tsp flaxseeds
2 tsp pumpkin seeds
1 tsp fructose
2 tsp flaked almonds

Place chopped nectarine in the bottom of a glass. Top with yogurt. Grind flaxseeds in blender, add pumpkin seeds and grind further. Mix the fructose and flaked almonds into the ground mix. Sprinkle on top of the yogurt and serve.

Warm Oat and Apple Bowl

Preparation: 5 minutes, Cooking: 5 minutes, Serves 1

Estimated GL per serving: 14

2 tsp olive or coconut oil
2 tbsp oats
1 tbsp sugar-free apple purée (or any other fruit variety)
2 tsp flaked almonds
2 tsp pumpkin seeds
2 tsp ground almonds
1 dsp natural, sugar-free yogurt

Heat the oil gently in a small saucepan. Add the oats and stir until starting to go golden. Add rest of ingredients and stir until heated through. Put in a bowl. Add yogurt on top and serve.

One-pot Wonders

One-pot Pork and Orange Casserole

Preparation: 15 minutes, Cooking: 35 minutes, Serves 4

Estimated GL per serving: 14

1 tbsp olive oil
1 large onion, chopped
1 clove garlic, crushed, or ½ tsp dried/purée
approx. 1 lb lean pork loin, cubed
1 tsp ground cumin
1¼ cups orange juice, with pulp
⅔ cup water
1 medium sweet potato, peeled and diced
2 medium carrots, peeled and chopped
1 small parsnip, peeled and chopped
1 tbsp arrowroot

Heat oil in a large saucepan. Fry onion, garlic and pork for 5 minutes. Add cumin and stir well. Add orange juice and water. Add the vegetables, cover and cook gently for about 30 minutes. Mix the arrowroot with 1–2 tbsp cold water and blend until smooth. Take the casserole off the heat and stir in the arrowroot. Keep on stirring—it should take less than a minute to thicken the sauce. Serve immediately.

Mediterranean Fish Stew

Preparation: 12 minutes, Cooking: 45 minutes, Serves 4–6

Estimated GL per serving: 2

2 tbsp olive oil

2 medium red onions, sliced

3 cloves garlic, crushed or grated

1 can (approx. 1½ cups) chopped tomatoes

approx. ½ cup organic vegetable stock

approx. ½ cup dry white wine

1 bay leaf

freshly ground black pepper

1.5 lb firm white fish fillets

2.2 lb mussels, cleaned

approx. 10 oz shrimp (fresh or frozen and thawed)

handful fresh parsley, chopped

Heat the oil in a pan and fry onions until softened. Add the garlic, tomatoes, half the stock, the wine, bay leaf and pepper and simmer for 15 minutes. Cut the fish into 2-inch squares, add to the pan and simmer for 15 minutes. Put the mussels into a large pan with the remaining stock, bring to a boil, cover and cook for 5 minutes until they have opened—discard any that have not. Add the mussels, with their liquid, and the shrimp to the main stew, cook for a further couple of minutes or until the shrimp are cooked. Pour into a serving dish, sprinkle with parsley and serve immediately.

Grilled Vegetable and Halloumi Pasta

Preparation: 15 minutes, Cooking: 10 minutes, Serves 4

Estimated GL per serving: 6

1 large zucchini, sliced

4 tomatoes, cut into quarters

1 bulb fennel, trimmed and sliced

1 red onion, sliced

1 packet halloumi cheese, cut into cubes

2 tbsp olive oil

2 garlic cloves, crushed or grated

1 tsp thyme (fresh or ½ tsp dried)

1 tsp rosemary (fresh or ½ tsp dried)

approx. 6 cups buckwheat pasta

1 tbsp Parmesan cheese, grated

fresh lemon wedges to serve with

Set grill to medium heat. Put all chopped veggies and the halloumi into a baking dish. Mix in olive oil, garlic, and herbs and toss all the ingredients well in the dish until well covered. Place under grill until nicely browned on all sides—take out and turn regularly, making sure the veggies and cheese don't burn. Cook the buckwheat pasta in a large saucepan of boiling water until just cooked but still firm to the bite (*al dente*) and drain well. Put the pasta back into the saucepan, add the veggies and halloumi plus any juices and stir well. Serve in individual bowls, sprinkled with Parmesan. Squeeze the lemon wedges for a bit of zing!

Summer Stir-fry

Preparation: 10 minutes, Cooking: 10 minutes, Serves 4

Estimated GL per serving: 2

2 tbsp peanut oil

1 red onion, sliced

3 garlic cloves, crushed or grated

1 tbsp fresh ginger, grated, or 1 tsp dried

4–6 baby carrots

1 red pepper, sliced

1 yellow pepper, sliced

3 celery sticks, chopped

1 cup cauliflower florets

1 cup broccoli florets

1 cup sugar snap peas or snow peas

1 cup beansprouts

4 tbsp soy sauce

2 tbsp dry sherry or dry white wine

freshly ground black pepper

Heat the oil in a wok or large frying pan. Add the onion, garlic and ginger and stir-fry for no more than 30 seconds. Add the carrots, peppers, celery, cauliflower, broccoli, sugar snaps and beansprouts and stir-fry for 3–4 minutes. Add the soy sauce, sherry and pepper and stir, frying for another minute. Serve immediately.

Veggie Gumbo

Preparation: 25 minutes, Cooking: 1 hour, Serves 4

Estimated GL per serving: 1

4 tbsp olive oil

1 eggplant

4 shallots, coarsely chopped

4 celery sticks, cut into chunks

2 tsp smoked paprika (normal paprika will work also)

½ tsp cayenne pepper

3 garlic cloves, crushed or grated

2 tbsp tomato purée

approx. 1½ cups chopped tomatoes

1 green pepper, cut into chunks

2 cups okra, thickly sliced (if you can't find okra, add a small
    sweet potato, peeled and cut into chunks, and a zucchini,
    cut into chunks)

½ small butternut squash, peeled and cut into chunks (or any
    squash or pumpkin)

2½ cups organic vegetable stock

Heat the oil in a large saucepan. Add the eggplant, shallots and celery and cook for 2–3 minutes. Stir in the paprika, cayenne pepper and garlic and cook for another minute. Add the tomato purée, tomatoes, the rest of the veggies and the stock and stir well. Bring to a boil, and then reduce to a simmer. Cover and cook for 1 hour, stirring occasionally.

Pumpkin Ratatouille

Preparation: 15 minutes, Cooking: 30 minutes, Serves 4

Estimated GL per serving: 3

4 tbsp olive oil

2 onions, chopped

3 garlic cloves, crushed or grated, or 1½ tsp dried or purée

1 tsp paprika

½ tsp ground allspice

1 eggplant, cut into chunks

approx. 3 cups pumpkin, deseeded, peeled and cut into
    chunks

1 red pepper, cut into chunks

1 yellow pepper, cut into chunks

approx. 1 cup tomatoes, skinned and chopped (or use drained
    canned whole tomatoes)

handful fresh parsley (optional)

1 tsp chopped fresh thyme or ½ tsp dried

freshly ground black pepper

Heat the oil in a large pan. Cook the onions in the pan over medium heat for about 5 minutes until softened. Stir in the garlic, paprika and allspice. Add the eggplant, pumpkin and peppers and cook until they start to soften—about 5 minutes. Stir in the tomatoes, herbs and pepper and cook for a further 15 minutes, stirring occasionally.

Delicious with the Herby Lemon Bulgur Wheat (page 209) as an accompaniment.

Lorraine's Chunky Veggie and Bean Soup

Preparation: 10 minutes, Cooking: 25–30 minutes, Serves 4

Estimated GL per serving: 18

1 tbsp olive oil

1 large onion, chopped

2 cloves garlic, finely diced or crushed

1 medium sweet potato, cubed

1 each yellow, green and red pepper (adds lovely color as well as flavor), cut into cubes or slices

2 celery sticks, sliced

2 carrots, diced or cubed

handful broccoli florets

handful mushrooms, sliced

1 tsp dried crushed chilies

2 tsp grated ginger root

2 cups kidney beans, drained and rinsed

2 cups chickpeas, drained and rinsed

5 cups organic vegetable stock

1 tbsp crème fraîche

freshly ground black pepper

Stir-fry onion and garlic until onions are soft. Add the rest of the vegetables, chilies, ginger root, beans, peas and stock and bring to boil. Simmer until veggies are softish, about 20 minutes. Fill a bowl with the bean soup and add the crème fraîche, grind over some black pepper to taste and ENJOY!

Fried Fish with Peppered Oat Crunch Crumb

Preparation: 5 minutes, Cooking time: 6 minutes, Serves 4

Estimated GL per serving: 2

handful fine oatmeal
freshly ground black pepper
4 fillets boneless white fish
1 free-range egg, beaten
2 tbsp peanut oil
sprinkling of malt vinegar

Put the oatmeal on a plate, grind over some black pepper and combine. Dip the fish in the beaten egg and coat thoroughly with the oatmeal. Heat the oil in a large heavy frying pan over a moderate–high heat. Fry the fish for about 3 minutes on each side, until it's cooked through and the oat crumb has turned golden and crispy. Serve with your choice of our recipes for "healthy" fries (see pages 181 and 182), plenty of vinegar and a side salad—mmm, enjoy your guilt-free fish and chips!

Sweet Potato Fries

Preparation: 5 minutes, Cooking: 15 minutes, Serves 4

Estimated GL per serving: 4

2 medium sweet potatoes
1 tbsp olive oil
freshly ground black pepper

Preheat oven to 350°F. Peel the sweet potatoes and cut into chunky fries. Brush with olive oil and grind over some black pepper. Place on a baking tray and bake for about 15 minutes or until slightly crisp on the outside and tender on the inside.

Great with the Fried Fish with Peppered Oat Crunch Crumb!

Selina's Rutabaga Fries

Preparation: 5 minutes, Cooking: 40 minutes, Serves 4

Estimated GL per serving: 10

2 rutabagas, peeled and cut into chunky fries
1 tbsp olive oil

Preheat oven to 350°F. Brush the rutabaga with the oil. Place on a baking tray and bake for about 40 minutes until slightly crisp on the outside but mouth-wateringly soft on the inside.

Great with our healthy fried fish recipe.

Roasted Vegetable Wedges

Preparation: 10 minutes, Cooking: 30–40 minutes, Serves 4

Estimated GL per serving: 14

1 small sweet potato, peeled and cut into chunky wedges

1 rutabaga, peeled and cut into wedges

4 new potatoes, washed and cut into wedges

1 carrot, peeled and cut into wedges

1 parsnip, peeled and cut into wedges

1 small beet, peeled and cut into wedges

4 tbsp peanut oil

Preheat oven to 350°F. Bring a pan of water to a boil and parboil all the veggies, except the beet, for a maximum of 5 minutes. Pick a baking tray large enough to take all the vegetable wedges in a single layer, pour the oil into the tray and put it in the oven until the oil sizzles. Drain the vegetable wedges well, put back in the saucepan, put on the lid and give them a good shake to fluff their outsides a little. Very carefully take the baking tray out of the oven. Put all the veggie wedges into the tray with the oil, turn to coat and put back into the oven for 30–40 minutes or until veggies have turned golden brown.

More Low-GL Dinners!

Olivia's Fabulous Meatballs

Preparation: 10 minutes, Cooking: 30 minutes, Serves 4

Estimated GL per serving: 0

1 red onion, roughly chopped

1 onion, roughly chopped

2 cloves garlic, peeled

1 zucchini, roughly chopped

approx. 1 lb lean minced pork

pinch turmeric

1 tsp cumin

1 tsp chili sauce

freshly ground black pepper

Put the onions, garlic and zucchini in a food processor and blitz (or grate them all). Place them and all other ingredients in a bowl and mix all together well. Form into balls and dry-fry in a pan for about 30 minutes, turning regularly.

These go really well with Olivia's Tomato and Roasted Red Pepper Sauce (see page 249).

Vegetable and Noodle Stir-fry

**Preparation: 5 minutes, Cooking: 5 minutes,
Serves 4 as a main dish**

Estimated GL per serving: 9

2 cups buckwheat noodles
3 tbsp peanut oil
1 large red onion, sliced
approx. 1 cup snow peas or sugar snap peas
approx. 1 cup beansprouts
1 clove garlic, chopped or grated or ½ tsp dried or purée
2 tbsp light soy sauce

To serve:
1 tbsp sesame seed oil or chili sauce
handful fresh cilantro, chopped, or 1 tsp dried

Cook the noodles as per the packet instructions until *al dente* or just cooked but not soft, then drain and rinse in cold water until cold and set aside. Heat the oil in a pan and, when very hot, add the onion, snow peas and beansprouts and stir-fry for about 1 minute. Stir in the garlic, then add the noodles and soy sauce and stir-fry together for another minute or so. Take off the heat and serve sprinkled with either sesame oil or chili sauce, depending on your taste. Sprinkle with fresh cilantro.

This is lovely with other veggies, too—peppers, zucchini or carrots.

Crustless Spinach Tart

Preparation: 5 minutes, Cooking: 15 minutes, Serves 4

Estimated GL per serving: 0

1 large bag fresh spinach, washed, drained (frozen spinach,
    thawed and drained, also works)

3 tbsp olive oil

1 medium onion, chopped

2 cloves garlic, chopped or grated, or 1 tsp dried or purée

1 tsp fresh thyme or ½ tsp dried

6 free-range eggs

1 tbsp Parmesan cheese, grated

1 tbsp mature Cheddar, grated

½ tsp grated nutmeg (optional)

freshly ground black pepper

Cook the spinach, with just the water left on the leaves after washing, for 6–8 minutes. Drain well in a sieve, pressing down on the spinach to get rid of any excess water. Chop the spinach finely. Put 1 tablespoon of the oil in a frying pan and cook the onion until translucent, stir in the garlic and thyme and add the spinach. Break the eggs into a bowl and stir in the cheeses, nutmeg and pepper. Heat the remaining oil in a medium pan, add the egg mixture and stir lightly until it begins to set. Cook for about 5 minutes until the underneath is set, then invert onto a plate, put a drop more oil in the pan, and slide it back, cooked side up, and cook until totally set.

Alternative fillings:

Sweet potato and red pepper; sweet potato, onion, mushrooms and mixed herbs; herbs and garlic; peppers and bacon.

This is lovely cold for the lunchbox.

Caroline's Fish Pie

Preparation: 15 minutes, Cooking: 20–30 minutes, Serves 2

Estimated GL per serving: 1

1 medium cauliflower
1 packet (approx. 9 oz.) smoked mackerel
approx. 1½ cups shrimp (fresh or frozen and defrosted)
juice of half a lemon
freshly ground black pepper
2 tbsp half-fat crème fraîche
1 cup milk
2 tsp creamed horseradish
2 tbsp grated cheese

Preheat oven to 350°F. Cut the cauliflower into chunks and boil until tender, then set aside in a colander to drain really well. Remove the skin from the smoked mackerel and flake it into an ovenproof dish. Be sure to remove any bones as you do so. Squeeze any excess water out of the shrimp, then sprinkle them over the fish. Squeeze over the lemon juice and add the black pepper. In a small saucepan, mix the crème fraîche, the milk and horseradish and gently warm through. Pour mixture over the fish. Mash the cauliflower with half the cheese and spread it over the fish. Sprinkle the rest of the cheese over the top of the cauliflower mash and grind over plenty of black pepper. Cook for about 20–30 minutes until nicely bubbling and browned on top.

Lesley's Albondigas Tonno (Tuna Balls)

Preparation: 10 minutes, Cooking: 10 minutes, Serves 2

Estimated GL per serving: 15

1 generous cup flaked tuna or boneless salmon or white fish
  (or a mixture of these)
1 free-range egg, beaten
¾ cup medium oatmeal
1 tbsp fresh parsley or herb of your choice
1 free-range egg, boiled and finely chopped
1 tbsp grated hard cheese
1 clove garlic, chopped or grated
freshly ground black pepper
extra oatmeal for coating
3 tbsp olive oil

Mix all ingredients except for olive oil, and extra oatmeal for coating, together thoroughly. Chill for 20–30 minutes. Roll into small walnut-size balls. Roll balls in the remaining oatmeal to coat thoroughly. Heat the olive oil in a pan over a medium heat and cook, stirring for 10 minutes, until cooked through and browned.

Serve with a homemade tomato sauce like Olivia's Tomato and Roasted Red Pepper Sauce (page 249), Simple Tomato Sauce (page 248) or a low-GL ready-made one.

Fennel and Ham "Barleyotto"

Preparation: 10 minutes, Cooking: 30–40 minutes, Serves 4

Estimated GL per serving: 4

2 tbsp olive oil–based spread

1 medium onion or 3 shallots, diced

2 large fennel bulbs, sliced thinly

2–3 cloves garlic, chopped or grated

approx. ½ cup dry white wine

1 cup pearl barley

approx. 3 cups organic chicken or vegetable stock

2 cups ham, cut into chunks

freshly ground black pepper

1 generous handful chopped parsley

1 tbsp fresh Parmesan cheese

Melt the olive oil-based spread in a large pan on medium heat. Add the onion and fennel and stir gently for about a minute, then add the garlic and cook for a further minute—don't let it burn. Pour in the wine to deglaze the pan, turn up the heat and bring to the boil. Boil for 4–5 minutes, stirring until it reaches the consistency of syrup. Turn down heat and add the barley. Add about one-third of the stock, stirring continuously. Once the stock is starting to be absorbed, pour in the rest of the stock and cook until it's all absorbed—about 30–40 minutes. Keep an eye on it and stir regularly. When the barley is within 5–10 minutes of being cooked, stir in the ham and grind over plenty of fresh black pepper, stir in well. Take off the heat and stir in the chopped parsley. Shave fresh Parmesan over the top.

Roasts

Roast Turkey

Preparation: 10 minutes, Cooking: 30 minutes, Serves 4

Estimated GL per serving: 0

1 large onion, cut into chunks
8 garlic cloves, peeled but left whole
4 skinless turkey breasts
1 tbsp olive oil
freshly ground black pepper
1 cup organic chicken or vegetable stock

Preheat oven to 350°F. Put the onion and garlic into a roasting tray. Rub the turkey breasts with a little olive oil and place on top of the onion and garlic in the tray. Add black pepper and pour in the stock. Cover the tray tightly with foil and roast for 30 minutes or until cooked through.

Roast Chicken Gorgonzola

Preparation: 10 minutes, Cooking: 25 minutes, Serves 4

Estimated GL per serving: 1

1 tbsp olive oil–based spread
4 free-range skinless chicken breasts
1 generous cup Gorgonzola or dolcelatte cheese, or similar
2 handfuls low-GL breadcrumbs (such as soy and flaxseed)
2 tbsp fresh mint, chopped, or 1 tsp dried or purée

Melt the spread in a large frying pan and cook the chicken breasts for 2 minutes. Transfer chicken to the oven and roast for about 20 minutes. Meanwhile, place the cheese in a bowl and mash using a fork. Stir in the breadcrumbs and mint and combine thoroughly. Remove chicken from oven and spread one side with cheese mixture. Return to oven and roast for 5 minutes or until chicken is thoroughly cooked through. Remove the roast chicken from oven, slice diagonally and serve.

Great with low-GL mash and veggies for Sunday lunch!

Perfect Roast Ham

Preparation: 20 minutes, Cooking: 3 hours, Serves 6

Estimated GL per serving: 2

4lb. 4 oz. lean piece of ham
water
1 medium carrot, cut into chunks
1 large onion, peeled and quartered
2 bay leaves
1 tbsp vinegar
1 tbsp agave syrup
1 tbsp grainy mustard

Place the ham in a saucepan, cover with clean cold water and bring to the boil. Allow to boil for 1 minute, then rinse the ham and the saucepan thoroughly under the cold tap to remove any excess salt. Cover with clean fresh water and add the carrot, onion, bay leaves, vinegar and agave. Bring to the boil, turn down the heat so that the water is barely simmering and leave to cook for 1 hour 40 minutes. Once cooked, take off the heat and leave to sit for 20–30 minutes in the cooking liquid. Heat the oven to 400°F. Take the ham out of the saucepan. Spread with the grainy mustard and place on a foil-lined tray. Roast for 20–30 minutes, until crispy and browned. Allow to rest for another 20–30 minutes before carving.

- Serve hot with your favorite low-GL veggies.
- Serve cold with a crunchy salad or use in wraps.

Nut and Vegetable Loaf

Preparation: 15 minutes, Cooking: 45 minutes, Serves 6

Estimated GL per serving: 4

2 cups nuts (walnuts, almonds, pecans, etc), finely chopped

5½ cups fresh low-GL breadcrumbs (sliced soy and flaxseed
   bread works well)

2 tbsp olive oil–based spread

2 onions, finely chopped

2 cloves garlic, chopped or grated

3 sticks of celery, finely chopped

1 large carrot, finely grated

1 generous cup cream cheese

1 tsp thyme (fresh or dried)

handful fresh parsley, finely chopped

3 large free-range eggs

freshly ground black pepper

Preheat oven to 350°F. Mix the nuts and breadcrumbs in a large bowl. Heat the olive oil in pan over a medium heat and cook the onions until soft. Stir in the garlic, then remove from heat. Put all ingredients into the bowl with the nuts and breadcrumbs and combine well—easiest to do this with your hands. Pack it well into a greased loaf tin and bake for 35–40 minutes until firm. Serve hot or cold.

Marvellous Mashes

Sweet Potato, Cauliflower and Minty Mash

**Preparation: 5 minutes, Cooking: 15 minutes,
Serves 6 as a side dish**

Estimated GL per serving: 6

1 small cauliflower, cut into quarters
1 clove garlic, chopped fine, or ½ tsp dried or purée
1 large sweet potato, peeled and cut into chunks
4 tbsp olive oil–based spread
large bunch fresh mint, chopped fine, or 1 tsp dried or purée
freshly ground black pepper

Put the cauliflower, garlic and sweet potato in a pan, steam or boil until they are tender. Drain and put back into the pan. Mash with the spread, then stir in the mint and pepper. Serve immediately.

Great with roasts and cold meats.

Carrot, Rutabaga and Coriander Mash

Preparation: 5 minutes, Cooking: 15 minutes, Serves 4 as a side dish

Estimated GL per serving: 9

4 large carrots, chopped into chunks
1 medium rutabaga, peeled and chopped into chunks
1 tsp ground cilantro
1 tsp olive oil–based spread

Boil the carrots and rutabaga in a large pan until tender; drain well. Mash with the spread and cilantro.

This makes a great topping for cottage pie.

Spicy Mashed Sweet Potato

**Preparation: 10 minutes, Cooking: 10 minutes,
Serves 4 as a side dish**

Estimated GL per serving: 10

4 small sweet potatoes
1 tsp garam masala
freshly ground black pepper
1 fresh red chili, deseeded and finely chopped (or pinch of hot
    chili powder or chili flakes)
2 tsp olive oil–based spread

Peel and chop the sweet potatoes into chunks, boil until
tender and drain. Stir in all the spices and mash with the
spread.

This can be made in advance and kept covered in a
warm oven—fluff with a fork when ready to serve.

Roasted Garlic and Rutabaga Mash

Preparation: 10 minutes, Cooking: 35 minutes, Serves 2

Estimated GL per serving: 14

2 whole bulbs garlic
1 large rutabaga
1 tsp olive oil–based spread
a few sprigs of thyme leaves

Roast the garlic whole on a baking tray in a hot oven for 20 minutes. Squeeze the garlic from the skin and set aside. In the meantime, peel and chop the rutabaga and boil in water for 10 minutes or until softened. Drain and mash with the roast garlic, spread and thyme.

Pea and Mint Mash

Preparation: 5 minutes, Cooking: 5 minutes, Serves 2

Estimated GL per serving: 5

2 cups frozen peas
1 tbsp crème fraîche
1 handful fresh mint, chopped, or 1 tsp dried or purée
1 tbsp extra virgin olive oil
freshly ground black pepper

Boil the peas until tender. Drain and put into a blender with the crème fraîche, mint and olive oil and blend until fairly smooth. Add pepper to taste and serve.

Mashed Parsnips with Black Pepper and Nutmeg

**Preparation: 10 minutes, Cooking: 5 minutes,
Serves 4 as a side dish**

Estimated GL per serving: 12

4 parsnips, peeled and cut into chunks
water
2 tsp olive oil–based spread
½ tsp ground nutmeg
freshly ground black pepper

Cover parsnips with water in a large saucepan and boil for about 5 minutes until just tender. Once cooked, drain really well. Mash with the spread and nutmeg. Add pepper to taste and serve.

Roasted Butternut Squash and Garlic Mash

Preparation: 5 minutes, Cooking: approx. 40 minutes, Serves 4 as a side dish

Estimated GL per serving: 0

1 large butternut squash
4 cloves garlic, whole and in their skins
1 tsp olive oil–based spread
freshly ground black pepper

Preheat oven to 350°F. Cut the squash in half and scoop out the seeds. Cut again, into 4 pieces. Place on a baking tray. Put a garlic clove on each piece of squash, cover loosely with foil and roast for 20–30 minutes or until tender. After about 20 minutes, remove the garlic cloves from the oven. Allow garlic cloves to cool slightly and then squeeze the pulp out and set aside. Once the squash is tender, take out of the oven and carefully scoop the flesh from the skin. Mash the squash, garlic and spread together. Add pepper to taste.

A Bit on the Side

Corn Fritters

**Preparation: 5 minutes, Cooking: 5 minutes,
Serves 4 (makes 8 fritters)**

Estimated GL per serving: 19

1 large free-range egg, beaten
1 tsp red curry paste
4 spring onions, finely sliced
1 red pepper, deseeded and diced
2 generous cups corn kernels
2 tsp soy sauce
¾ cup medium oatmeal
1 tbsp olive oil

Beat the egg and curry paste together. Add onions, pepper, corn and soy sauce. Stir in the oatmeal. Shape into 8 round fritter shapes. Heat oil in a pan and fry for 2 minutes each side.

Roast Red Onion and Beet Wedges

Preparation: 5 minutes, Cooking: 20 minutes, Serves 4

Estimated GL per serving: 2

4 medium cooked beets, cut into wedges
2 large red onions, cut into wedges
1 tbsp olive oil
2 tbsp balsamic vinegar or pomegranate juice

Preheat oven to 400°F. Place beets and onions on a baking tray. Cover with olive oil and vinegar or juice. Roast for 20 minutes and serve.

Stir-fried Brussels Sprouts

Preparation: 5 minutes, Cooking: 5 minutes, Serves 4

Estimated GL per serving: 0

1 tsp olive oil
1 garlic clove, chopped, or ½ tsp dried or purée
3 cups Brussels sprouts, sliced
1 tsp olive oil–based spread
2 tbsp flaked almonds
squeeze of fresh lemon juice

Heat oil in a pan and stir-fry the garlic and Brussels sprouts for a few minutes until sprouts are cooked through. Add spread and almonds and stir. Add a squeeze of lemon juice and serve.

Onion Bhajis

**Preparation: 10 minutes, Cooking: 10 minutes,
Serves 4 as a side dish/starter**

Estimated GL per serving: 7

¾ cup gram flour

2 tsp cumin seeds

1 tsp ground cilantro

1 tsp turmeric

½ tsp mixed spice

4 tbsp water

1 large onion, finely chopped

1 sweet potato, grated

4 tbsp olive oil

Mix together the gram flour and all spices. Add water to
make a smooth batter. Add sliced onions and grated
sweet potato and mix well. Heat oil in a heavy-based
frying pan and gently drop in spoonfuls of the mixture.
Cook until golden brown on all sides. Remove from oil
and drain before serving.

Chinese Sugar Snap Peas

**Preparation: 5 minutes, Cooking: 5 minutes,
Serves 4 as a side dish**

Estimated GL per serving: 1

3 tbsp groundnut (peanut) oil
4 cups sugar snap peas (or snow peas)
4 spring onions, sliced on the slant
2 garlic cloves, chopped or grated
2 tbsp soy sauce
3 tbsp organic vegetable stock or water

Heat the oil in a wok or deep frying pan. Add the sugar snaps and stir-fry over high heat for about 1 minute. Add the spring onions and garlic and stir-fry for another minute. Turn down the heat, and add the soy sauce and stock. Stir well and serve.

Herby Lemon Bulgur Wheat

**Preparation: 5 minutes, Cooking: 15 minutes,
Serves 4 as a side dish**

Estimated GL per serving: 5

1½ cups bulgur wheat
zest and juice of 1 lemon
handful fresh cilantro
handful fresh parsley
few sprigs of lemon thyme
1 tbsp extra virgin olive oil

Cook the bulgur wheat as per the packet instructions. Once cooked, drain thoroughly and squeeze out any excess water. Grate the lemon zest finely into the bulgur wheat and squeeze over the lemon juice. Chop the herbs very fine and stir through the bulgur wheat, along with the olive oil. Serve warm or cold.

Green Beans and Basil

**Preparation: 5 minutes, Cooking: 10 minutes,
Serves 4 as a side dish**

Estimated GL per serving: 0

1 tbsp pine nuts
1 tbsp extra virgin olive oil
1 shallot, finely chopped
3 cups French beans
1 tsp lemon juice
handful fresh basil
freshly ground black pepper
1 tbsp fresh Parmesan cheese
pine nuts

Bring a pan of water to a boil for the beans. Toast the pine nuts in a dry pan until golden; set aside. Use the warm pan to heat the oil and gently fry the shallot for a few minutes. Meanwhile, boil the beans for about 5 minutes, until just starting to become tender. Drain well and transfer into a warmed serving bowl. Stir the lemon juice into the cooked shallots. Pour over the beans and toss well. Sprinkle with pine nuts, basil and black pepper, toss again. Shave over some Parmesan and serve.

Andie's Rostis

Preparation: 5 minutes, Cooking: 5 minutes, Serves 1

Estimated GL: 21

3 spring onions, finely chopped
1 small sweet potato, grated
1 zucchini, grated
1 large carrot, grated
1 free-range egg, beaten
2 tbsp gram flour
2 tsp olive oil

Mix all ingredients together. Heat olive oil in a pan and fry until golden brown on both sides.

Olivia's Salmon Rosti Topping

Make Andie's Rostis as above. Top each one with a generous strip of smoked salmon and a poached egg. Drizzle a little olive oil over the top, and garnish with some chopped chives.

Sexy Salads

Walnut and Goat's Cheese

Preparation: 6 minutes, Serves 2

Estimated GL per serving: 0

1 bag mixed salad leaves
½ cup walnut halves
1 cup goat's cheese, cubed
1 tbsp balsamic vinegar
1 tbsp walnut oil
freshly ground black pepper

Wash and dry the salad leaves. Place into a bowl with the walnuts and goat's cheese. Drizzle over the vinegar and oil, toss with black pepper and serve immediately.

Melon and Anchovy

Preparation: 10 minutes, Serves 2

Estimated GL per serving: 7

1 small melon
small bag salad leaves, washed and dried
4 anchovy fillets
juice of half a lemon
juice of half an orange

Halve the melon and scoop out the seeds. Cut the melon flesh into cubes and put into a serving dish. Add the salad leaves. Drain the anchovy fillets, but keep a table-spoon of the oil. Cut them into slivers and add to the salad. Mix the lemon and orange juice with the anchovy oil and pour over the salad.

Feta and Beets

Preparation: 5 minutes, Serves 2

Estimated GL per serving: 8

4 whole cooked beets, cut into wedges

1 tbsp walnut oil (can use other nut oils or olive oil)

2 tsp white wine vinegar

1 tsp grainy mustard

small bag mixed leaves

½ cup feta cheese, crumbled

⅛ cup walnuts, toasted

Combine all ingredients, toss together and serve.

Grilled Pears with Blue Cheese and Watercress

Preparation: 5 minutes, Cooking: 3 minutes, Serves 2

Estimated GL per serving: 4

2 pears, firm and ripe
½ cup blue cheese, cubed
2 handfuls watercress, washed and drained
freshly ground black pepper

Cut the pears in half and carefully remove the core. Fill the pear halves with the blue cheese, put under a very hot grill for a couple of minutes until cheese melts. Divide the watercress between two plates. Place two pear halves on top of the watercress on each plate. Grind over black pepper and serve immediately.

Chickpea Salad

Preparation: 5 minutes, Serves 4

Estimated GL per serving: 6

approx. 2 generous cups chickpeas, drained and rinsed
2 tsp cumin
2 garlic cloves, chopped, or 1 tsp dried or purée
juice of 2 lemons
1 red onion, finely chopped
1 tbsp extra virgin olive oil
pinch cayenne pepper
2 tbsp fresh parsley, chopped
freshly ground black pepper

Combine all ingredients together in a bowl.

Good to make in advance and keep in the fridge overnight to allow the flavors to infuse.

Watercress Tabbouleh

Preparation: 20 minutes, Cooking: 10 minutes, Serves 2

Estimated GL per serving: 2

½ cup bulgur wheat
1 large bag watercress, washed, drained and finely chopped
handful fresh mint, finely chopped
juice and zest of 1 lemon
2 tbsp extra virgin olive oil
3 tomatoes, finely chopped
6 spring onions, finely chopped

Add the bulgur wheat to a pan of boiling water and simmer for 10 minutes. Drain in a sieve and cool with running cold water. Squeeze to remove excess water. In a serving bowl combine the bulgur wheat, watercress and mint. Add all remaining ingredients and mix well.

Allow the flavors to infuse for an hour in the fridge before serving.

Wraps

Sally's Cajun Chicken Wrap

Preparation: 10 minutes, Cooking: 10 minutes, Serves 4

Estimated GL per serving: 12

2 skinless, boneless chicken breasts
2 tbsp olive oil
2 tsp Cajun spice mix
4 tbsp half-fat crème fraîche
handful fresh chives, chopped
4 stoneground wholemeal tortilla wraps
half an iceberg lettuce
8 cherry tomatoes, halved
half a cucumber, sliced

Chop the chicken breasts and fry in the oil on a moderate heat for about 10 minutes until they start to brown. Add the Cajun spice mix and coat the chicken thoroughly. Mix the crème fraîche and the chives in a bowl. Spread each tortilla wrap with the crème fraîche mixture. Place some lettuce, tomatoes and cucumber on each wrap and top with a quarter of the Cajun chicken. Roll the wraps.

Crunchy Veggie Wrap

Preparation: 7 minutes, Serves 1

Estimated GL per serving: 11

1 avocado, peeled and pitted
2 sundried tomatoes, chopped
dash of Tabasco or other pepper sauce
squeeze of lemon juice
1 stoneground wholemeal tortilla wrap
handful bean sprouts
handful iceberg lettuce, shredded
freshly ground black pepper

Mash the avocado, sundried tomatoes and Tabasco together. Squeeze in a little lemon juice to taste. Place the avocado mash on the tortilla, then the beansprouts and lettuce, and pepper to taste, and roll the wrap.

Goat's Cheese, Sundried Tomato and Arugula Wrap

Preparation: 5 minutes, Serves 1

Estimated GL per serving: 10

2 tbsp soft goat's cheese
4 sundried tomatoes, chopped fine
1 stoneground wholemeal tortilla wrap
1 handful arugula, washed and dried

Mash the goat's cheese and tomatoes together. Spread the goat's cheese on the wrap. Add the arugula on top and roll the wrap.

Grilled Veggie Wrap

Preparation: 15–20 minutes, Serves 2

Estimated GL per serving: 12

1 zucchini, sliced

1 red onion, sliced

1 red pepper, sliced

1 tbsp olive oil

1 tbsp balsamic vinegar

1 clove garlic, chopped (optional)

freshly ground black pepper

1 small handful pine nuts

1 handful fresh basil or 1 tsp dried basil

2 tbsp hummus

1 stoneground wholemeal tortilla wrap

Preheat the grill to a high heat. Put the vegetables onto a baking tray in a single layer. Add the olive oil, vinegar and garlic, and toss to ensure all well covered. Grind over black pepper and place under the grill for about 5 minutes or until golden brown, being careful not to burn. Toss, sprinkle with pine nuts and put back under the grill for 2 minutes. Spread the hummus on the wraps, add the veggies and the basil and roll the wraps. Serve immediately.

Prawn Cocktail Wrap

Preparation: 5 minutes, Serves 1

Estimated GL per serving: 10

handful cooked frozen shrimp (thoroughly defrosted and
    dried)
1 tbsp mayonnaise
1 tsp tomato ketchup
1 tsp paprika
1 handful shredded lettuce
1 stoneground wholemeal wrap

Mix the prawns, mayonnaise, ketchup and paprika
together. Place the lettuce on the wrap. Spread the
mixture on top and roll the wrap.

Snacks and Dips

Dipping Sticks!

Estimated GL per serving: 0

The following savory dips and spreads make great, healthy snacks to keep hunger at bay. Make up your favorite healthy "dipping sticks" every day so they are always at hand for snacking:

- Carrot sticks (you can also buy ready-washed, sweet baby carrots from the supermarkets)
- Cucumber sticks
- Pepper sticks (green, orange, red and yellow—each has its own unique taste!)
- Celery sticks

Halloumi Cheese Slices

Slice the cheese and fry in olive oil, then eat hot or cold as a snack, or add to salads. Use two slices as a snack.

Add herbs and spice for variety.

Seedy Cinnamon Mix

Cooking: 10 minutes

Estimated GL per serving: 0

1 handful each of your favorite seeds: pumpkin, sunflower,
    flaxseed, sesame, etc.
1 tsp ground cinnamon

Add seeds to a large dry frying pan with the cinnamon
and "toast" over a high heat until the seeds start to turn
golden. Turn down the heat and keep them moving in
the pan so they do not burn. Allow to cool and store in
an airtight jar.

Both nuts and seeds have a low GL *but* are high in
calories, so just a small handful in total of either nuts or
seeds (or a mix of both) per day if you are in weight-loss
mode.

Choco Craving Drink

Preparation: 5 minutes, Serves 1

Estimated GL per serving: 2

2 heaped tsp cocoa (sugar-free)
2 tsp agave syrup
mug of your choice of milk
sugar-free aerosol whipped cream

To sprinkle:
Cocoa (sugar-free) and fructose (mixed half and half in a
shaker)

Mix the cocoa in the base of a mug with the agave syrup,
add a splash of cold water and blend well until smooth
(you can buy tiny mini-whisks that are great for this).
Boil the milk in a pan and gradually stir it into the cocoa
mix in the mug, mixing thoroughly. Top with whipped
cream and sprinkle with the cocoa-and-fructose mix.

Keep your cocoa-and-fructose mix in a plastic shaker
to shake over the top of your hot chocolate or latte.

Keep a shaker with cinnamon powder and fructose in
too, for a change.

Yummy Egg Slices

Preparation: 5 minutes, Cooking: 5 minutes, Serves 1

Estimated GL per serving: 0

1 free-range egg, boiled
Your choice of the following toppings:
    cream cheese, sprinkled with paprika
    hard cheese slices, topped with a small amount of mayo
      and a slice of tomato
    shrimp, cucumber and marie rose sauce
    hummus and celery

Cut the egg into three chunky slices and spread each slice with your chosen topping.

A very filling snack!

Egg and Sundried Tomato Bowl

Preparation: 5 minutes, Serves 1

Estimated GL per serving: 0

1 free-range egg, hard-boiled and chopped
1 tsp mayonnaise
1 tsp chopped cucumber
1 tsp sundried tomato

Mix all together in a ramekin.

Baba Ganoush

Preparation: 5 minutes, Cooking: 4 minutes, Serves 4

Estimated GL per serving: 0

3 tbsp extra virgin olive oil
2 eggplant, diced
2 garlic cloves, peeled
juice of 1 lemon
4 tbsp fresh basil

Heat the oil in a frying pan and cook the eggplant until soft. Blend eggplant and all other ingredients in a food processor until they form a rough paste.

A great healthy spread or dip.

Avocado Hummus

Preparation: 10 minutes, Serves 4

Estimated GL per serving: 5

approx. 2 cups chickpeas, drained
1 ripe avocado
1 crushed garlic, or ½ tsp garlic powder/purée
juice of 1 lemon
freshly ground black pepper
pinch paprika

Blend the chickpeas, avocado and garlic in a blender.
Add lemon juice, black pepper and paprika and mix well.
Nice spread on oatcakes or low-GL toast.

Sardine and Tomato Bowl

Preparation: 5 minutes, Serves 2

Estimated GL per serving: 0

1 can sardines in tomato sauce
dash Tabasco or other pepper sauce
dash Worcestershire sauce
a few sprigs fresh basil, chopped (optional)

Empty the sardines with sauce into a bowl. Add the Tabasco, Worcester sauce and basil, mash with a fork and mix well.

A good way to eat your oily fish portion at least once a week!

Avocado Snack

Preparation: 5 minutes, Serves 1

Estimated GL per serving: 0

half an avocado, peeled and pitted
1 tsp lemon juice
freshly ground black pepper
pinch garlic powder

Mash or blend all ingredients together.

Tuna Snack

Preparation: 5 minutes, Serves 2

Estimated GL per serving: 0

1 medium can tuna, drained
half a red onion, chopped
2 tsp balsamic vinegar
2 tsp mayonnaise

Mash or blend all ingredients together.

Hummus Snack

Preparation: 5 minutes, Serves 1

Estimated GL: 1

1 tbsp hummus
quarter of a red pepper, chopped
pinch paprika

Combine or blend all together.

Fruity Yog-bowls

Preparation: 5 minutes, Serves 1

Estimated GL: 5

2 tsp sugar-free fruit purée
1 tbsp natural, sugar-free yogurt
1 swirl sugar-free aerosol whipped cream

Spoon the sugar-free fruit purée into a ramekin. Spoon yogurt on top. Add a swirl of sugar-free whipped cream on top.

"Sugar-free" fruit purées are a great "fast-and-friendly" low-GL snack; you can use them in recipes when you need fruit or a bit of natural sweetness. They come in choices such as apple, apple / strawberry, apple / orange, apple / blueberry, and apple / apricot, and are portable so don't need to be kept refrigerated. See our website for retailers.

Cheesy Avocado Dip

Preparation: 5 minutes, Serves 1

Estimated GL: 0

half a ripe avocado, peeled and pitted
2 tsp cream cheese
freshly ground black pepper
squeeze of lemon juice

Mash or blend all ingredients together.

Beanie Dip

Preparation: 5 minutes, Cooking: 5 minutes, Serves 2

Estimated GL per serving: 2

1 clove garlic, chopped, or ½ tsp dried or puréed

1 small red onion, chopped

1 tsp olive oil

half an eggplant, chopped

1 tbsp tomato purée

approx. ½ cup butter beans, drained

freshly ground black pepper

Sauté garlic and onion in hot oil until softened. Add eggplant and cook until golden brown. Add tomato purée, butter beans and black pepper and stir-fry for 1 minute. Blend all ingredients together briefly—leave chunky.

Avocado Salsa

Preparation: 5 minutes, Serves 2

Estimated GL per serving: 0

1 avocado, peeled, pitted and diced
2 large tomatoes, diced
1 small red onion, finely chopped
handful fresh cilantro or ½ tsp dried
juice of 1 lime (or lemon)
freshly ground black pepper

Place all ingredients in a bowl and combine.

Butter Bean and Herb Dip

Preparation: 5 minutes, Serves 4 as a dip

Estimated GL per serving: 5

1 can/2 cups butter beans, drained and rinsed
4 tbsp natural, sugar-free yogurt
juice of half a lemon
pinch of paprika
pinch of cayenne pepper
1 garlic clove, chopped
2 tbsp extra virgin olive oil
small handful fresh basil leaves
freshly ground black pepper

Add all ingredients together and blend until smooth. If you prefer it chunky, just pulse lightly until roughly chopped.

Red Pepper Dip

Preparation: 15 minutes, Cooking: 5 minutes, Serves 4

Estimated GL per serving: 0

2 tbsp extra virgin olive oil

1 shallot, sliced

1 clove garlic, chopped

1 red pepper, deseeded and chopped

1 tsp chili powder

Heat the olive oil in a small pan. Add all the ingredients. Fry for about 5 minutes. Blend all ingredients together until smooth.

Lentil and Bacon Dip

Preparation: 15 minutes, Serves 4 as a dip

Estimated GL per serving: 4

2 cups lentils, cooked
1 tsp Worcestershire sauce
8 rashers lean bacon, grilled and roughly chopped
2 tbsp extra virgin olive oil
1 tsp white wine vinegar
pinch chili
freshly ground black pepper

Combine all ingredients and blend until smooth.

Sauces and Dressings

Olive and Anchovy Dressing

Preparation: 5 minutes, Serves 2

Estimated GL per serving: 0

large handful pitted green olives
2 anchovy fillets
1 clove garlic, chopped
1 tbsp lemon juice
1 tbsp extra virgin olive oil

Place all ingredients in a blender and blend until smooth.

Makes a lovely dressing for grilled or poached fish.

Hot Salsa Dressing

Preparation: 10 minutes, Cooking: 5 minutes, Serves 4

Estimated GL per serving: 0

2 tbsp olive oil

3 tomatoes, chopped into chunks

2 shallots, chopped

1 garlic clove, finely chopped

½ tsp chili powder

1 tbsp balsamic vinegar

1 tsp lemon juice

Heat the olive oil in a pan. Add the tomatoes, shallots, garlic and chili powder and fry for 5 minutes. Take off the heat and stir in the vinegar and lemon juice.

Delicious with fish, grilled meat, or as a warm salad dressing. Also very nice cold.

Garlic and Mustard Dressing

Preparation: 5 minutes, Serves 4

Estimated GL per serving: 0

1 tsp mustard of your choice
1 clove garlic, finely chopped or grated
1 tsp lemon juice
3 tbsp extra virgin olive oil
1 tbsp white wine vinegar
freshly ground black pepper

Combine all ingredients together in a blender and blend until smooth.

Salsa Verde

Preparation: 5 minutes, Serves 4

Estimated GL per serving: 0

1 tbsp mustard of your choice
1 tsp freshly ground black pepper
2 cloves garlic, chopped
1 shallot, chopped
handful fresh herbs (i.e. tarragon, parsley, chives, cilantro or
    dill) or a sprinkling of dried herbs
3 tbsp white wine vinegar
4 tbsp extra virgin olive oil
2 free-range eggs, hard-boiled

Combine all ingredients and blend, or finely chop eggs first and then mix all ingredients together well if not using a blender.

Lovely with poached or grilled fish, hot or cold beef, and green beans.

French Dressing

Preparation: 7 minutes, Serves 4

Estimated GL per serving: 0

1 clove garlic, finely chopped

1 tbsp lemon juice

2 tsp Dijon mustard

4 tbsp extra virgin olive oil

freshly ground black pepper

Mix the garlic, lemon juice and mustard in a bowl. Slowly whisk in the oil until creamy. Add black pepper to taste. Blend or shake together in a jar.

Two-Minute Fresh Herb Sauce

Preparation: 2 minutes, Cooking: 2 minutes, Serves 2

Estimated GL per serving: 0

2 tbsp crème fraîche
1 tsp olive oil–based spread
1 tbsp fresh herbs, finely chopped (choose from parsley,
    cilantro, thyme, rosemary, chives)
freshly ground black pepper

Heat the crème fraîche gently in a pan with the spread.
Stir in the herbs and black pepper and serve.

Great with fish or pasta.

Simple Tomato Sauce

Preparation: 5 minutes, Cooking: 10 minutes, Serves 2

Estimated GL per serving: 1

2 tbsp olive oil

3 garlic cloves, crushed or grated

2 cups chopped tomatoes

¾ cup tomato passata (sieved tomatoes—you can buy in jars
    or cartons at the grocery store)

1 tsp balsamic vinegar

2 dashes Tabasco sauce (optional)

3 dashes Worcestershire sauce (optional)

handful fresh basil, chopped roughly or 1 tsp dried basil

freshly ground black pepper

Heat the oil in a frying pan, add the garlic and cook gently until soft. Add the chopped tomatoes, passata, vinegar, Tabasco and Worcestershire. Bring to a boil quickly, stirring continuously. When the sauce has thickened, stir in the basil and black pepper before serving.

Great for pasta and all fish and meat dishes.

Olivia's Tomato and Roasted Red Pepper Sauce

Preparation: 15 minutes, Cooking: 15 minutes, Serves 2

Estimated GL per serving: 1

1 tbsp olive oil

1 onion, chopped

1 garlic clove, chopped

1 red pepper, cut into sections, grilled until the skin is black
    and blistered—peeled and sliced

approx. 2 cups chopped tomatoes

1 cup water

1 tbsp tomato purée

1 tbsp sundried tomato purée (optional)

1 tsp cayenne pepper (optional)

freshly ground black pepper

Heat the oil in a pan, add onion and garlic and cook until they are gently softened. Add the red pepper and heat for another minute. Add the rest of the ingredients. Bring to the boil and simmer for approximately 10 minutes. Either serve as is or blend for a smoother sauce.

You can change the herbs to use the sauce with different dishes.

Fast Gravy

Preparation: 6 minutes, Cooking: 5 minutes, Serves 2

Estimated GL per serving: 1

1 cup organic vegetable, chicken or beef stock
1 tsp arrowroot

Put 1 tablespoon of the stock in a cup, blend thoroughly with the arrowroot and set aside. Place the rest of the stock in a pan on the stove and start to heat. Pour in arrowroot mixture and stir or whisk until it thickens. Remove the stock from the heat as soon as it has boiled.

If you buy organic stock, it won't contain hydrogenated/trans fats as many of the non-organic ones do.

Sweet Sauces

Orange Custard

Preparation: 10 minutes, Cooking: 6 minutes, Serves 4

Estimated GL per serving: 5

2½ cups your choice of milk
grated zest of 1 orange
8 free-range egg yolks
3 tbsp fructose
1 tsp arrowroot powder

Bring the milk to just below boiling point in a pan with the orange zest, but don't boil. Beat the egg yolks and fructose in a bowl until really light and fluffy—almost mousse-like. Pour the milk over the egg-and-fructose mix, stirring all the time. Rinse and dry the milk pan. Pour the custard mixture back into the pan and place on a low heat. Mix the arrowroot with 1 tablespoon of cold water to make a smooth paste, then stir or whisk into the custard. Take off the heat and stir until it thickens.

To make vanilla custard, replace the orange zest with a teaspoon of good-quality vanilla extract.

Chocolate Drizzle Sauce

Preparation: 2 minutes, Serves 4

Estimated GL per serving: 2

2 tbsp sugar-free cocoa
2 tbsp agave syrup

Combine using a mini-hand whisk or a blender.

Use chilled for a "treat" topping for ice cream, yogurt or oatmeal.

Apple Compote

Preparation: 5 minutes, Cooking: 10 minutes, Serves 2

Estimated GL per serving: 6

2 large apples
2 tsp fructose or agave syrup
1 tsp ground ginger
1 tsp nutmeg
3 tbsp water

Peel and core the apples and slice into a small saucepan. Add the fructose, ginger and nutmeg and stir. Pour over the water and put on a low–medium heat on the stove, bring to the boil, turn down and cover with a lid. Cook for 10 minutes on a low heat, stirring and making sure it doesn't burn.

Serve hot or cold.

Goes well with yogurt or added to oatmeal, or as a topping for vanilla ice cream.

Desserts

Ginger and Kiwi Fruit Salad

**Preparation: 10 minutes (plus an hour to infuse),
Serves 4**

Estimated GL per serving: 12

1 medium-size melon, cut in half and deseeded
2 kiwis (not over-ripe), peeled and thinly sliced
2 cups mixed seedless grapes, cut in half
½ tsp ground ginger or 1 tsp freshly grated ginger
6 tbsp apple juice (fresh rather than made from concentrate)

Cut the melon flesh into cubes, or use a melon baller. Place in a bowl with the kiwi fruit and grapes. Mix the ginger and apple juice together. Pour over the fruit and leave in the fridge for an hour to infuse before serving.

Black Currant Brûlée

**Preparation: 5 minutes, Cooking: 10 minutes,
Cooling: 1 hour, Serves 4**

Estimated GL per serving: 0

approx. 4 cups black currants, washed and stalks removed
1 tbsp water
1 tbsp agave syrup or fructose
½ cup natural, sugar-free yogurt

For topping:
1 tbsp fructose
1 tbsp flaked almonds

Put the black currants in a pan with the water and cook until soft. Add the agave syrup or fructose and stir. Divide the fruit between 4 heatproof ramekins and put in the fridge to chill thoroughly. Preheat grill to a moderate temperature. Spoon the yogurt on top of the fruit and sprinkle with the fructose and almonds. Place ramekins under the grill until the fructose has melted and the almonds are golden brown. Serve immediately.

- You can use any other berries.
- You can use crème fraîche in place of the yogurt.

Pomegranate Muffins

Preparation: 5 minutes, Cooking: 5–15 minutes (depending on cooking method), Serves 4

2 tbsp olive oil–based spread, melted

2 large free-range eggs

approx. 1 generous cup ground almonds

1 tbsp pomegranate seeds

1 tsp baking powder

1 tbsp fructose or agave syrup

1 tbsp pomegranate juice

If baking in the oven, preheat to 375°F. Whisk the melted spread and eggs together. Add rest of ingredients and mix all together thoroughly. Spoon a tablespoon of the mix into 4 individual microwaveable ramekin dishes and microwave for about 1 minute each or until springy on top. Alternatively, bake muffins in a medium oven in a non-stick muffin tin for about 15 minutes. Whichever cooking method you choose, be careful not to over-cook—the muffins are ready when light and springy on top.

Pomegranate and ginger go well together, so you might want to add a teaspoon of powdered or grated fresh ginger.

You can adapt and play with this recipe to make other flavored muffins by taking out the pomegranate seeds and juice and replacing them with:

- a handful of chopped strawberries, raspberries, blueberries, apple, apricot, pear or peach (add a pinch of cinnamon if using apple)
- 1-7 oz. of 70 percent-plus cocoa dark chocolate, broken into small pieces
- 2 teaspoons lemon or orange oil and 1 teaspoon of lemon or orange zest.

Grilled Ginger Pineapple

Preparation: 5 minutes, Cooking: 5–7 minutes, Serves 2

Estimated GL per serving: 16

1 small fresh pineapple, peeled and sliced, or a small can of
    slices in natural juice with no added sugar (not in syrup)
1 tsp olive oil spread, melted
½ tsp dried ginger
1 dsp agave syrup
½ tsp ground cinnamon

Arrange slices of pineapple on a foil-lined baking tray and brush with the melted spread. Mix the ginger with the agave syrup and cinnamon and spread over the pineapple slices. Place under a hot grill for 5–7 minutes until golden brown.

Summer Fruit Compote with Greek Yogurt

Preparation: 20 minutes, Serves 4

Estimated GL per serving: 2

approx. 4 cups summer berries (fresh or frozen)
1 tbsp agave syrup or fructose
4 tbsp Greek yogurt
handful toasted pine nuts or flaked almonds

Put the berries into a saucepan and gently heat, squashing them with a wooden spoon, for about 5 minutes. Put berries in a bowl, add the agave or fructose, stir together and set aside for about 10 minutes for flavors to combine. Spoon the yogurt into 4 individual serving dishes. Spoon over the fruit mixture, sprinkle with the nuts and serve.

Baked Rhubarb Crumble

Preparation: 10 minutes, Cooking: 30 minutes, Serves 4

Estimated GL per serving: 12

approx. 6 cups rhubarb, washed, prepared and cut into 1-inch
    pieces
1 tbsp agave syrup or fructose
1 tsp fresh ginger, grated or ½ tsp dried
grated zest of 1 orange
juice of 1 orange

For the crumble:
approx. 1 cup oats
⅔ cup ground almonds
2 tbsp crushed walnuts
grated zest of 1 lemon
2 tsp fructose
2 tbsp olive oil–based spread
handful flaked almonds for topping

Preheat oven to 350°F. Pack the rhubarb into a baking dish, drizzle over the agave syrup, stir in ginger and orange zest and pour over the orange juice. For the crumble, combine the oats, almonds, walnuts, lemon zest and fructose in a bowl. Use clean hands to add the spread, making a crumble with your fingertips. Sprinkle the crumble topping over the rhubarb. Sprinkle over the flaked almonds and bake in the oven for up to 30 minutes, checking regularly to make sure the top doesn't burn.

Rhubarb freezes well raw or cooked.

Fruity Cheese Plate

Preparation: 10 minutes, Serves 4

Estimated GL per serving: 10

1½ oz (matchbox-size serving) blue cheese, cut into chunky
     slices
1½ oz Jarlsberg cheese or similar, cut into chunky slices
1½ oz seedless grapes, halved
1½ oz fresh raspberries
1 pear, ripe but firm, cored and cut into wedges
8 sugar-free oatcakes
1 tbsp olive oil–based spread in a ramekin to spread on
     oatcakes

Arrange all attractively on a large serving plate and help
yourself.

Melting Chocolate Pudding

Preparation: 20 minutes, Cooking: 15 minutes, Serves 4

Estimated GL per serving: 5

6 tbsp olive oil–based spread

approx. 1½ cups dark chocolate (70 percent-plus cocoa),
    broken into pieces

2 free-range eggs

2 free-range egg yolks

3 tbsp fructose

⅔ cup ground almonds

Preheat oven to 325°F. Grease 4 ramekins or individual pudding molds. Place the olive oil spread and the chocolate pieces into a heat-proof bowl. Place the bowl over a pan of simmering water and allow chocolate to melt slowly (or carefully melt it for about 1 minute in a microwaveable bowl in the microwave, but take care it does not burn). Stir and leave to cool. Add eggs and egg yolks to a bowl. Add fructose and whisk until it's pale and thick and the mixture leaves a trail on top. Fold in the chocolate mix and gradually fold in the ground almonds. Divide into the 4 ramekins and bake for 12 minutes or until set. Remove from oven and either serve in the ramekins or run a knife around the edge of the ramekin and turn out to serve.

Top with sugar-free whipped cream or, for a special treat, a scoop of vanilla ice cream.

Flapjacks

Preparation: 5 minutes, Cooking: 15 minutes, Serves 8

Estimated GL per serving: 10

5 tbsp olive oil–based spread

1 tbsp agave syrup

1 cup fructose

⅔ cup oats

⅔ cup ground almonds

1 cup desiccated coconut (sugar-free)

Preheat oven to 350°F. Grease a medium-size square baking tray. Melt olive oil–based spread in a large saucepan with the agave syrup. Stir over a low heat until melted. Remove from heat and stir in fructose, oats, almonds and coconut, and mix well. Turn the mixture into the baking tray and spread evenly. Bake for 15 minutes, remove from oven and carefully cut into squares while still hot. Allow to cool completely before removing from tray.

Baked Apple Custard

Preparation time: 10 minutes, Cooking time: 30 minutes, Serves 2

Estimated GL per serving: 6

2 medium free-range eggs
1 tbsp fructose
⅔ cup natural, sugar-free yogurt
1 tsp arrowroot
1 tsp natural vanilla extract
1 apple, cored and sliced thinly

Preheat oven to 325°F. Whisk all ingredients except for apple together until smooth. Divide apple slices into the bases of 2 heat-proof ramekins. Pour custard mix over the top. Bake in oven for 30 minutes or until custard is set and golden on top.

Quick-bake Cinnamon Cakes

Preparation: 5 minutes, Cooking: 15 minutes, Serves 4

Estimated GL per serving: 2

1 free-range egg
just 1 cup ground almonds
2 tsp cinnamon
1 tbsp fructose
1 tsp baking powder

Preheat oven to 350°F. Beat egg well. Mix all dry ingredients together, making sure you mix the baking powder in well. Fold into the egg. Spoon into paper bun cases or into a muffin tin. Bake for up to 15 minutes. Allow to cool before serving.

Alternatives:

To make coconut buns, add 1 oz. of dessicated coconut (sugar-free), or you can replace 1 oz. of the ground almonds with 1 oz. of oatmeal for a different texture. You can also use this basic recipe without the fructose and flavorings to make savory "cakes"—try adding grated cheese and mustard or sundried tomatoes!

Chocolate and Almond Torte

This is only for a very special treat or celebration!

Preparation: 15 minutes, Cooking time: 1 hour, Serves 8

Estimated GL per serving: 10

1⅓ cups olive oil–based spread
2 cups fructose
4 cups 70% cocoa dark chocolate
6 free-range eggs
2½ cups roast almonds, roughly ground

Preheat oven to 375°F. Beat the fructose and spread together until creamy. Melt the chocolate in a bowl over boiling water, not letting the bowl touch the water, or melt carefully for 20 seconds or so in the microwave, taking care it does not burn. Stir the melted chocolate into the fructose and spread mixture. Beat the eggs for about a minute. Fold the beaten eggs into the chocolate-and-fructose mixture. Stir in the roasted almonds. Pour mixture into a 8- or 9-inch pastry ring and bake for up to 1 hour until cooked through.

A–Z OF LOW-GL FOODS

We have included a list of our recommended low-GL foods for extra guidance. The list contains only healthy, low-GL foods (no jam doughnuts or sausage rolls in sight!). We have listed an average portion size and, for tested foods, the GL value. If foods haven't been tested yet, but we assume that they will have a low GL based on similar foods, we have included them (you will see NT, which stands for "not tested," in the GL column). Foods that contain either no carbohydrate or only a minimal amount, we have listed as 0 in the GL column. The 0 foods will have no glycemic impact.

More foods are being tested for their GL value all the time, including many branded goods. If you would like to keep up to date with newly tested low-GL foods and products, visit our website at www.dietfreedom.co.uk.

You can use the food list along with the recipes in this book to help you keep your daily GL total low. A low daily GL is classed as 80 GL or less, and a high GL is 120 GL or higher. We have included only low-GL foods on the list: low-GL foods have a GL value of 10 or less per portion.

You can use this as a guide, but don't get too hung up on counting (it's boring), just focus on "swapping" high-GL foods for low-GL foods—it's easy once you get started and will become second nature very quickly. If you want to lose weight rather than just eat healthily, swap to low-GL foods and keep an eye on your portion sizes. You can do this easily by using the "cupped hands" method of not eating any more at each meal (based on three meals a day) than you can fit into your cupped hands.

PLEASE NOTE: If foods are normally eaten cooked, the weights given are cooked weights, unless otherwise stated.

A

	Average portion	GL
Agave Syrup	10g	2
Anchovies*	120–150g	0
Apple	120g	5
Apple juice	125ml	6
Arrabiata sauce	2–3 tbsp	NT
Artichoke	80g	0
Asparagus	80g	0
Avocado	80g	0
Avocado, mint and lime dressing	1 tbsp	NT

B

Baked beans	80g	4
Balti sauce	2–3 tbsp	NT
Banana (green—under-ripe)	60g	3

	Average portion	GL
Banana (yellow and green)	60g	6
Banana (ripe)	60g	7
Bean sprouts	80g	NT
Beef	75–120g	0
Beets	80g	4
Black-eyed peas	80g	5
Black pepper sauce	2–3 tbsp	NT
Blackberries	120g	0
Black currant	120g	0
Blueberries	120g	0
Blueberry juice	125ml	7
Bolognese sauce	2–3 tbsp	NT
Bran sticks (sugar-free)	30g	NT
Broccoli	80g	0
Brown rice	75g	9
Brussels sprouts	80g	0
Buckwheat kasha (boiled)	100g	10
Bulgur wheat (boiled)	100g	8
Butter	20g	0
Butter beans	80g	3

C

Cabbage	80g	0
Caesar dressing	1 tbsp	NT
Carrot juice	125ml	5
Carrots	80g	2
Cashews	50g	3
Cauliflower	80g	0
Caviar	1 tbsp	0
Celery	80g	0

	Average portion	GL
Celery Root (Celeriac)	80g	0
Chana dal	80g	2
Cheese—all types	50–75g	0
Cheese and chive dip	1 tbsp	NT
Cheese and onion dip	1 tbsp	NT
Cheese sauce	2–3 tbsp	NT
Cherries	120g	3
Chicken	100–150g	0
Chickpeas	80g	4
Chili dressing	1 tbsp	NT
Chocolate—choose chocolate containing at least 70 percent cocoa. A few squares as a snack is a great healthy choice!	20g (2 squares)	NT
Cocoa	10g	NT
Coffee—be aware that some coffee bar chains add syrups to their coffees, which will make them high-GL—ask for plain coffee or a cappuccino.	1 cup	0
Coleslaw	1 tbsp	0
Collard greens	80g	0
Corn	80g	9
Couscous	100g	7
Cranberry juice	125ml	8
Cream	1 tbsp	NT
Crème fraîche	2 tbsp	NT
Cucumber	80g	0

D

Dark Swiss rye bread	30g	9
Diet drinks	1 can/bottle	0

	Average portion	GL
Dried apple	60g	10
Dried apricot	60g	9
Dried peach	60g	8
Dried prunes	60g	6
Duck	100–150g	0

E

	Average portion	GL
Eggplant	80g	0
Eggs	1	0
Endive	80g	0

F

	Average portion	GL
Falafel	100g	NT
Fava beans	80g	5
Fettuccine (egg-based pasta)	100g	10
Figs (fresh)	120g	NT
Flaxseed	50g	NT
French dressing	1 tbsp	NT
Fructose	10g	2
Fruit tea	unlimited	NT

G

	Average portion	GL
Game	100–150g	0
Garlic and herb dip	1 tbsp	NT
Goat's milk	125ml	NT
Grapefruit	120g	1–3
Grapefruit juice	125ml	4–6
Grapes—black	120g	10
Grapes—green	120g	8
Guacamole	1 tbsp	NT

	Average portion	GL
H		
Haricot (navy) beans	80g	6
Hazelnuts	50g	NT
Hemp seeds	50g	NT
Herbal tea	unlimited	NT
Herrings*	120–150g	0
Honey	25g	10
Honey and mustard dressing	1 tbsp	NT
Hummus	100g	<1
I		
Ice cream (plain vanilla)	50g	3–8
J		
Jam (jelly), reduced sugar	30g	5
K		
Kale	80g	0
Kidney	75–120g	0
Kidney beans	80g	5
Kippers*	120–150g	0
Kiwis	120g	6
Kohlrabi	80g	0
Korma sauce	2–3 tbsp	NT
L		
Lamb	75–120g	0
Leeks	80g	0
Lemons	1	0

	Average portion	GL
Lentils	80g	3
Lettuce (all types)	80g	0
Lima beans	80g	5
Limes	1	0
Liver	75–120g	0

M

	Average portion	GL
Macadamia nuts	50g	NT
Mackerel*	120–150g	0
Madeira sauce	2–3 tbsp	NT
Madras (curry) sauce	2–3 tbsp	NT
Mandarins	120g	NT
Mangoes	120g	8
Maple syrup	25g	9
Mayonnaise	1 tbsp	NT
Melons	120g	4
Milk, cow's (max total milk per day 284ml)	125ml	2
Muesli (sugar free)	30g	7–16
Mung bean noodles, dried	100g	8
Mung beans	80g	5
Mushroom sauce	2–3 tbsp	NT
Mushroom (Forestière) sauce	2–3 tbsp	NT
Mushrooms	80g	0

N

	Average portion	GL
Napoletana sauce	2–3 tbsp	NT
Nectarines	120g	NT

	Average portion	GL
O		
Oat bran (raw)	10g	3
Oat bran and honey bread	30g	7
Oatcakes	30g	8
Oats (steel-cut, cooked in water)	30g (dry weight)	9
Okra	80g	0
Olive oil	1 tbsp	0
olive oil–based spread	20g	0
Olives	80g	0
Onions	80g	0
Orange juice	125ml	5
Oranges	120g	5
Ostrich	100–150g	0

	Average portion	GL
P		
Papaya	120g	9–10
Parsnips	80g	8
Peaches	120g	5
Peanuts	50g	1
Pearl barley	100g	5
Pears	120g	4
Peas	80g	3
Peas (marrowfat)	80g	4
Peas (split yellow)	80g	3
Pecans	50g	NT
Peppers	80g	0
Pesto sauce	2–3 tbsp	NT
Pine nuts	50g	NT
Pineapple juice	125ml	8

	Average portion	GL
Pineapples	120g	7
Pinto beans	80g	5
Pistachio nuts	50g	NT
Plums	120g	5
Pomegranate juice	125ml	12
Popcorn (plain, microwaved)	20g	8
Pork	75–120g	0
Potatoes (baby new)	80g	6
Prunes (pitted)	60g	10
Pumpernickel bread	30g	5
Pumpkin	80g	3
Pumpkin seeds	50g	NT
Puttanesca sauce	2–3 tbsp	NT

Q

Quinoa, organic, boiled	100g	9
Quorn	100–150g	NT

R

Radicchio	80g	0
Radishes	80g	0
Raspberries	120g	0
Ravioli	100g	8
Red pepper dressing	1 tbsp	NT
Red wine and herb sauces	2–3 tbsp	NT
Rhubarb	120g	0
Rice bran, extruded	30g	3
Rice noodles	100g	10
Roasted vegetable sauces	2–3 tbsp	NT

	Average portion	GL
Runner beans	80g	0
Rutabaga	80g	7
Rye (whole)	30g (dry weight)	8
Rye crackers	30g	10

S

	Average portion	GL
Salmon* (canned or fresh)	120–150g	0
Sardines*	120–150g	0
Sauerkraut	80g	0
Sausages (choose 90% meat)	75–120g	0
Semolina (steamed)	100g	4
Sheep's milk	125ml	NT
Shellfish	120–150g	0
Shrimp	120-150g	0
Snow peas	80g	0
Soba (buckwheat) noodles	100g	NT
Sour cream	1 tbsp	0
Sour cream and chive dip	1 tbsp	NT
Sourdough rye bread	30g	6
Soy (meat alternative)	100–150g	NT
Soy and flaxseed bread	30g	3
Soybeans	80g	<1
Soy milk	125ml	2
Soy yogurt	100g	6
Spaghetti, white	100g	10
Spaghetti, wholemeal	100g	9
Spelt hasn't been individually tested so use sparingly for now.		
Spelt multigrain bread	30g	7

	Average portion	GL
Spinach	80g	0
Spinach and ricotta or nutmeg sauce	2–3 tbsp	NT
Spring onions (scallions)	80g	0
Squash (all)	80g	0
Strawberries	120g	1
Sunflower and barley bread	30g	6
Sunflower seeds	50g	NT
Sweet pepper sauce	2–3 tbsp	NT
Sweet potatoes	80g	9
Swiss chard	80g	0

T

	Average portion	GL
Tabbouleh	50g	NT
Tangerines	120g	NT
Tarragon sauce	2–3 tbsp	NT
Tea (black/green)	unlimited	NT
Tikka masala sauce	2–3 tbsp	NT
Tomato and basil dressing	1 tbsp	NT
Tomato and basil sauce	2–3 tbsp	NT
Tomato and mascarpone sauce	2–3 tbsp	NT
Tomato and roasted onion dressing	1 tbsp	NT
Tomato juice	125ml	2
Tomato salsa	1 tbsp	NT
Tomatoes	80g	0
Tortellini, cheese	100g	6
Tuna*	120–150g	0
Turkey	100–150g	0
Turnips	80g	0
Tzatziki	1 tbsp	NT

	Average portion	GL
U		
Ugli fruit	120g	NT
V		
Vinaigrette dressing	1 tbsp	NT
W		
Walnuts	50g	NT
Watercress	80g	0
Watercress sauce	2–3 tbsp	NT
Watermelon	120g	4
Wheat (whole)	30g (dry weight)	8
White fish	150–200g	0
White wine sauce	2–3 tbsp	NT
Whole-grain bread	30g	7
Wholemeal pita bread	30g	10
Wholemeal rye bread	30g	8
Wild rice	75g	8
Y		
Yams	80g	7
Yogurt	200g	2–4
Yogurt and mint dressing	1 tbsp	NT
Yogurt drinks (sugar-free)	1 standard size	NT

	Average portion	GL
Z		
Zucchini	80g	0

denotes oily fish

	Day 1	Day 2	Day 3	Day 4	Day 5	Day 6	Day 7
Breakfast							
Mid-morning Snack							
Lunch							

	Day 1	Day 2	Day 3	Day 4	Day 5	Day 6	Day 7
Mid-afternoon Snack							
Dinner							

(You can also print this blank plan from our website.)

FURTHER HELP AND SUPPORT

Our website www.dietfreedom.co.uk is an online resource for all things GL and health related.

You can join our online **Diet Freedom Members' Club** to gain access to the following exclusive services:

"Ask the Dietician"

Personal and confidential responses to your questions direct to your inbox, plus a database of FAQs. We keep our members up to speed on all things GL and health related including the latest tested foods.

Forums

Our lively forums provide a great support network with members from all over the world. It's fun, friendly and inclusive—we as authors post regularly. It is our inspiration, and the feedback we receive is of huge importance to us.

One-to-Ones

If you need a bit more emotional support with your weight issues, we provide either face-to-face or phone consultations with our team of qualified registered dieticians. Members receive a discount on all services.

Food Lists

Members have access to our *Low-GL-Food List* and portion guide, which is updated with newly tested foods.

Recipe Database

We have an extensive database that contains hundreds of low-GL recipes.

Newsletter

Our fortnightly members' e-mailed newsletter keeps you up to speed on all things GL, with GL success stories, latest GL research, competitions and offers, and lots of chat.

RECOMMENDED RETAILERS

Although you can easily follow a low-GL diet without buying special foods, you can visit www.dietfreedom.co.uk for a list of retailers for any of the recommended low-GL alternative ingredients mentioned that may be difficult to find. For example:

- agave syrup
- buckwheat flour
- buckwheat pasta
- dark chocolate
- fructose
- gram flour
- oat flour
- oatmeal
- products with no added sugar
- quinoa flour
- spelt flour

Appendix 3

RECOMMENDED READING

Denby, Nigel, Michelucci, Tina and Pyner, Deborah, *The 7-Day GL Diet* (Harper Thorsons Element, 2005)

Denby, Nigel, Michelucci, Tina and Pyner, Deborah, *The GL Diet Cookbook* (Harper Thorsons Element, 2006)

Denby, Nigel, Michelucci, Tina and Pyner, Deborah, *The GL Diet Made Easy* (Harper Thorsons Element, 2006)

Denby, Nigel, *The GL Diet* (John Blake, 2004)

Denby, Nigel, *Nutrition for Dummies* (Hungry Minds, 2005)

Denby, Nigel and Baic, Sue, *The GL Diet for Dummies* (Wiley, 2006)

Rinzler, Carol Ann, *Nutrition for Dummies* (Wiley, 2005)

Index

Index of Recipes

Other Ulysses Press Books

The Easy GL Diet Handbook: Lose Weight with the Revolutionary Glycemic Load Program

Dr. Fedon Alexander Lindberg, $10.00

Using these more accurate and sensible GL scores, *The Easy GL Diet Handbook* offers a plan for healthy weight loss and reduced risk of diabetes that's easier to follow. It also includes numerous foods that the Atkins, South Beach, and GI diets wrongly consider "off-limits."

The Leptin Boost Diet: Unleash Your Fat-Controlling Hormones for Maximum Weight Loss

Scott Isaacs, M.D., $14.95

A series of recent medical breakthroughs have confirmed what physicians suspected all along—obesity is a hormonal disorder. *The Leptin Boost Diet* transforms these findings into a unique and easy-to-follow weight-loss program that is perfect for people whose out-of-balance hormones make it impossible to lose weight on other diets.

The Simple 0-to-10 GI Diet: Lose Weight with the Easy Food Scoring System Based on the Glycemic Index

Azmina Govindji & Nina Puddefoot, $12.95

Balancing blood glucose by eating the right carbs is vital to losing weight, but the glycemic index's complicated scoring system makes it difficult to keep track of total carb intake. By simplifying the scoring system and creating an easy-to-follow plan, this book offers a no-hassle program to lose weight and maintain a healthy long-term diet.

Mastering Cortisol: Stop Your Body's Stress Hormone from Making You Fat around the Middle

Marilyn Glenville, $15.95
Details specific ways to counter cortisol with a tailor-made exercise plan that will slim the belly. Based on breakthrough genetic tests, the program also recommends specific vitamins and minerals and explains which foods will work best for the reader.

Prediabetes Wake-Up Call: A Personal Road Map to Prevent Diabetes

Beth Ann Petro Roybal, $14.95
Includes assessment checklists and charts to identify areas of relative risk, and details specific strategies to address each risk factor.

Weight-Bearing Workouts for Women: Exercises for Sculpting, Strengthening & Toning

Yolande Green, $12.95
Weight training is the fastest, most effective way to lose fat, improve muscle tone and strengthen bones. This workbook shows just how easy it is for women at any age to get started with weights.

To order these books call 800-377-2542 or 510-601-8301, fax 510-601-8307, e-mail ulysses@ulyssespress.com, or write to Ulysses Press, P.O. Box 3440, Berkeley, CA 94703. All retail orders are shipped free of charge. California residents must include sales tax. Allow two to three weeks for delivery.

About the Authors

Nigel Denby, RD BSc Hons, is a UK–based state registered dietician specializing in obesity and women's health. He runs a diabetes clinic within the UK National Health service and has his own private practice in London. Nigel regularly appears on UK television including BBC's *Real Story* and ITV's *Trevor McDonald Tonight*.

Tina Michelucci and **Deborah Pyner** are co-founders of www.dietfreedom.co.uk, a supportive online health and diet club. Both are passionate patient advocates and, as ex-serial dieters, have great empathy and understanding on all diet and health-related issues. Tina previously set up and ran a successful health and leisure complex while Deborah previously worked in marketing. They now run Diet Freedom, writing content and recipes as well as developing the Diet Freedom food product range, which includes delicious low-GL, gluten-free cakes. See www.dietfreedom.co.uk for more information. If you'd like to join the club, enter the code GLDME when prompted to obtain a 20 percent discount.